Osteoporosis

Natalie E. Cusano
Editor

Osteoporosis

A Clinical Casebook

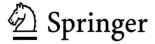 Springer

Editor
Natalie E. Cusano
Division of Endocrinology
Lenox Hill Hospital
New York, NY
USA

ISBN 978-3-030-83950-5   ISBN 978-3-030-83951-2   (eBook)
https://doi.org/10.1007/978-3-030-83951-2

This Springer imprint is published by the registered company Springer Nature
Switzerland AG
The registered company address is: Gewerbestrasse 11, 6330 Cham, Switzerland

Preface

Osteoporotic fractures are expected to increase with the aging of the population, causing a significant stress on healthcare systems worldwide. Despite noninvasive methods for screening and highly effective therapies, osteoporosis remains underdiagnosed and undertreated. The first report on the disease from the United States Office of the Surgeon General stated that bone health was "critically important" for overall health and well-being. The consequences of osteoporotic fractures are excess mortality, morbidity including total or partial disability, loss of independence, and impaired quality of life, in addition to economic costs.

This book is designed to aid in the management of osteoporosis through a patient-focused approach. The authors have related clinical pearls from their extensive backgrounds to address some of the challenges providers face in the treatment of osteoporosis. I would like to acknowledge the contributors for sharing their experience, and hope that this book assists the reader in reducing the burden of the disease for their patients, male and female, and across the age spectrum.

New York, NY, USA   Natalie E. Cusano, MD, MS

Contents

Contributors

Robert A. Adler Endocrinology and Metabolism Section, Central Virginia Veterans Affairs Health Care System and Division of Endocrinology, Metabolism, and Diabetes, Virginia Commonwealth University, Richmond, VA, USA

Valerie S. Barta Division of Nephrology, Lenox Hill Hospital, Donald and Barbara Zucker School of Medicine at Hofstra/Northwell, New York, NY, USA

John P. Bilezikian Division of Endocrinology, Vagelos College of Physicians and Surgeons, Columbia University, New York, NY, USA

Joanne Bruno Division of Endocrinology, Diabetes, and Metabolism, Department of Medicine, New York University Langone Medical Center, New York, NY, USA

Pauline Camacho Division of Endocrinology, Loyola University Osteoporosis and Metabolic Bone Disease Center, Loyola University Medical Center, Maywood, IL, USA

Cristiana Cipriani Department of Clinical, Internal, Anesthesiological and Cardiovascular Sciences, Sapienza University of Rome, Rome, Italy

Bart L. Clarke Mayo Clinic E18-A, Rochester, MN, USA

Natalie E. Cusano Division of Endocrinology, Lenox Hill Hospital, New York, NY, USA

Maria V. DeVita Division of Nephrology, Lenox Hill Hospital, Donald and Barbara Zucker School of Medicine at Hofstra/Northwell, New York, NY, USA

Katherine Haseltine Hospital for Special Surgery, New York, NY, USA

Steven W. Ing Division of Endocrinology, Diabetes and Metabolism, The Ohio State University Wexner Medical Center, Columbus, OH, USA

Sumeet Jain Division of Endocrinology, Rush University Medical Center, Chicago, IL, USA

Bente L. Langdahl Department of Endocrinology and Internal Medicine, Aarhus University Hospital, Aarhus, Denmark

E. Michael Lewiecki New Mexico Clinical Research & Osteoporosis Center, Albuquerque, NM, USA

Emilia Pauline Liao Northwell Health Lenox Hill Hospital, New York, NY, USA

Priyanka Majety Division of Endocrinology, Diabetes and Metabolism, Beth Israel Deaconess Medical Center, Boston, MA, USA

Alan Ona Malabanan Division of Endocrinology, Diabetes and Metabolism, Beth Israel Deaconess Medical Center, Boston, MA, USA

Harvard Medical School, Boston, MA, USA

Brinda Manchireddy Endocrinology and Metabolism Section, Central Virginia Veterans Affairs Health Care System and Division of Endocrinology, Metabolism, and Diabetes, Virginia Commonwealth University, Richmond, VA, USA

Maria Gabriela Negron Marte Endocrinology and Metabolism Section, Central Virginia Veterans Affairs Health Care System and Division of Endocrinology, Metabolism, and Diabetes, Virginia Commonwealth University, Richmond, VA, USA

Swetha Murthi Northwell Health Lenox Hill Hospital, New York, NY, USA

Jordan L. Rosenstock Division of Nephrology, Lenox Hill Hospital, Donald and Barbara Zucker School of Medicine at Hofstra/Northwell, New York, NY, USA

Laura E. Ryan Division of Endocrinology, Diabetes and Metabolism, The Ohio State University Wexner Medical Center, Columbus, OH, USA

Parinya Samakkarnthai Robert and Arlene Kogod Center on Aging, Mayo Clinic, Rochester, MN, USA

Jad G. Sfeir Robert and Arlene Kogod Center on Aging, Mayo Clinic, Rochester, MN, USA

Division of Endocrinology, Diabetes, Metabolism, and Nutrition; Division of Geriatric Medicine and Gerontology, Mayo Clinic, Rochester, MN, USA

Barbara C. Silva Endocrinology Division, Felicio Rocho Hospital, Belo Horizonte, Brazil

Endocrinology Division, Santa Casa Hospital, Belo Horizonte, Brazil

Department of Medicine, Centro Universitario de Belo Horizonte (UNI-BH), Belo Horizonte, Brazil

Maria Marta Sarquis Soares Endocrinology Division, Felicio Rocho Hospital, Belo Horizonte, Brazil

Department of Medicine, Federal University of Minas Gerais (UFMG), Belo Horizonte, Brazil

Jessica Starr Hospital for Special Surgery, New York, NY, USA

Clinical Medicine, Weill Cornell Medical College, New York, NY, USA

New York Presbyterian Hospital, New York, NY, USA

Melissa Sum Division of Endocrinology, Diabetes, and Metabolism, Department of Medicine, New York University Langone Medical Center, New York, NY, USA

Guido Zavatta Mayo Clinic E18-A, Rochester, MN, USA

Abbreviations

25OHD	25-hydroxyvitamin D
95% CI	95% confidence interval
BMI	Body mass index
BMD	Bone mineral density
CT	Computed tomography
DXA	Dual energy X-ray absorptiometry
eGFR	Estimated glomerular filtration rate
EMA	European Medicines Agency
FSH	Follicle stimulating hormone
FDA	Food and Drug Administration
FRAX	Fracture risk assessment tool
HR	Hazard ratio
IV	Intravenous
IU	International units
LH	Luteinizing hormone
OR	odds ratio
PTH	Parathyroid hormone
PO	per os/by mouth
RANK	Receptor activator of κB
RANKL	Receptor activator of κB ligand
RR	Relative risk
SC	Subcutaneous
TSH	Thyroid stimulating hormone

Challenges in Screening and Diagnosis of Osteoporosis

1

Natalie E. Cusano

Case Presentation

A 69-year-old man with a history of coronary artery disease and rheumatoid arthritis on prednisone was referred for hyperparathyroidism secondary to vitamin D deficiency. For his rheumatoid arthritis, he was treated with hydroxychloroquine and had been on and off prednisone for the past 10 years, most recently 5 mg daily for the past 6 months. Bone density testing was recommended since he had no history of previous evaluation and was significant for T-scores of −0.2 at the lumbar spine, −2.2 at the femoral neck, and −1.7 at the total hip. Degenerative changes were noted at the lumbar spine. Vertebral fracture assessment demonstrated a T12 compression fracture. He had no history of trauma, and spine imaging 5 years prior was without fracture.

He was diagnosed with glucocorticoid-induced osteoporosis in the setting of an atraumatic vertebral fracture, despite densitometric osteopenia. Metabolic evaluation for secondary causes of bone loss was remarkable for calcium 9.8 mg/dL (albumin 4.2 g/dL; normal: 8.4–10.5), PTH 98 pg/mL (normal: 15–65),

N. E. Cusano (✉)
Division of Endocrinology, Lenox Hill Hospital, New York, NY, USA
e-mail: ncusano@northwell.edu

25-hydroxyvitamin D 14 ng/mL, and BUN/creatinine 12/0.84 mg/dL (eGFR >60 mL/min). Testosterone, serum/urine protein electrophoresis, and transglutaminase antibody testing were within range. 24-hour urine calcium was not obtained at that time due to vitamin D deficiency.

He was counseled regarding calcium intake of 1200 mg from diet and supplements in divided doses. His vitamin D deficiency was addressed with ergocalciferol 50,000 IU weekly for 3 months, with recommendation for 1000 IU daily subsequently. Pharmacologic osteoporosis treatment options were discussed.

Assessment and Diagnosis

Osteoporosis is defined as a skeletal disorder characterized by compromised bone strength predisposing to an increased risk of fracture [1]. The word is derived from "osteo-" pertaining to bone + the Greek stem "poros" meaning "passage" or "pore," literally, "porous bone." This is easily visualized from bone specimens of patients with osteoporosis versus individuals with healthy bone. With osteoporosis, cortical bone, the outer shell of bone, is thinner; there are also fewer trabecular struts, and the trabeculae are thinner, leading to a porous appearance (Fig. 1.1).

Using data obtained from the National Health and Nutrition Examination Survey (NHANES), in 2010, an estimated 10.2 million Americans had osteoporosis and 43 million had low bone mass [2]. In 2005, there were over 2 million osteoporotic fractures in the USA: 547,426 vertebral fractures, 296,610 hip fractures, 296,961 wrist fractures, and over 800,000 fractures at other sites [3]. There were an estimated 9 million fractures worldwide in 2000, and across the world, 1 in 3 women over 50 and 1 in 5 men will experience an osteoporotic fracture [4]. For a 50-year-old woman, her estimated lifetime risk of death from a hip fracture is 2.8%, equal to her risk of death from breast cancer [5].

A fragility fracture is a fracture occurring from a low energy trauma that would not ordinarily result in fracture. The WHO has quantified a fragility fracture to occur from a force equivalent to a fall from standing height or less [6]. Osteoporosis is often called

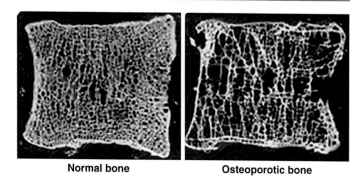

Normal bone **Osteoporotic bone**

Fig. 1.1 Comparison of a vertebral bone specimen from an individual with healthy bone (left) compared to a patient with osteoporosis (right), demonstrating a porous appearance due to effects including decreased trabecular number and thickness. (Permission to use image granted by Turner Biomechanics Laboratory)

a "silent disease" because there are no symptoms until a fracture occurs. Major osteoporotic fractures are defined as fractures of the spine, hip, distal radius, and proximal humerus, although osteoporotic fractures can also occur in the ribs, pelvis, and other bones. Fractures at certain sites, including the skull, cervical spine, hands, feet, and ankles, are not generally considered to be fragility fractures.

Fractures lead to significant morbidity and mortality. Approximately 20% of patients will die in the year following a hip fracture and up to 90% will have difficulty with at least one activity of daily living 1 year after fracture [7, 8]. Fractures also lead to significant healthcare costs, with $19 billion spent in 2005 and $25.3 billion projected by 2025 [3]. For these reasons, early diagnosis and initiation of effective therapy are key in the management of osteoporosis.

It is preferable to make a diagnosis of osteoporosis in a patient prior to the occurrence of fracture through noninvasive screening. Dual-energy X-ray absorptiometry (DXA) is the standard of care to diagnose osteoporosis, assess fracture risk, and monitor treatment response. The accuracy and precision of DXA are excellent [9]. A typical DXA machine consists of a padded table for the

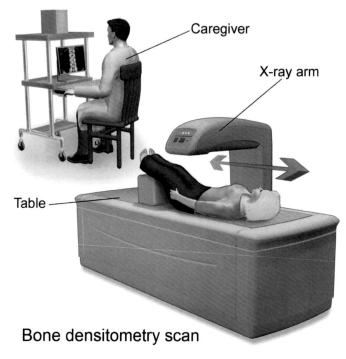

Bone densitometry scan

Fig. 1.2 A typical DXA machine with demonstration of patient positioning for the lumbar spine scan

patient to lie on, a radiograph tube below the patient, and a detector above the patient (Fig. 1.2) [10]. Bone and soft tissue have different attenuation coefficients to X-rays. DXA uses two separate energies of X-rays (thus, "dual energy"). The difference in total absorption between the two separate energies can be used to subtract out the absorption by soft tissue, leaving the absorption by bone. DXA measures bone mineral content (BMC, in grams) and bone area (BA, in square centimeters). By dividing BMC by BA, areal BMD in g/cm^2 is obtained. The risk to the patient from radiation exposure from DXA is very low, overall equivalent to daily background radiation [9]. Pregnancy remains a contraindication for DXA due to the risks of ionized radiation.

Table 1.1 WHO definition of osteoporosis based on BMD measurements by DXA*

Definition	BMD measurement	T-score
Normal	BMD within 1 SD of the mean bone density for young adults	T-score ≥ -1.0
Low bone mass (osteopenia)	BMD 1–2.5 SD below the mean for young adults	T-score between -1.0 and -2.5
Osteoporosis	BMD ≥ 2.5 SD below the normal mean for young adults	T-score ≤ -2.5
Severe/"established" osteoporosis	BMD ≥ 2.5 SD below the normal mean for young adults in a patient who has already experienced ≥ 1 fractures	T-score ≤ -2.5

*Applicable to peri-/postmenopausal women and men ≥ 50 years

In 1994, the WHO classified bone density according to standard deviation (SD) differences between an individual's BMD and that of a young-adult reference population, termed a T-score [6]. Low bone mineral density (BMD) is a powerful predictor of fracture risk. For each SD decline in bone density, fracture risk increases twofold. The WHO definitions are as follows (Table 1.1): T-score ≥ -1.0 is normal, T-score -1.1 to -2.4 is osteopenia, and T-score ≤ -2.5 is osteoporosis. The National Osteoporosis Foundation (NOF) and the International Society for Clinical Densitometry (ISCD) recommend the WHO criteria be applied to the lowest T-score site among the posteroanterior lumbar spine (L1–L4), femoral neck, and total hip [11, 12]. Of note, BMD at the lumbar spine site can be falsely elevated in the setting of degenerative disease. Measurement of the distal 1/3 radius is recommended by the ISCD if the lumbar spine or hip sites are not able to be measured due to the presence of hardware or are otherwise uninterpretable, for patients with primary hyperparathyroidism due to a preferential risk for cortical bone loss, or in patients with body weight above the limits of the table [12].

The WHO classifications can be used for postmenopausal women and men ≥ 50 years [12]. For younger women and men, a diagnosis of osteoporosis cannot be made by bone density alone since the relationship between BMD and fracture risk is not well established in younger patients. A diagnosis of osteoporosis in younger patients may be made in the presence of a fragility fracture, or when there is low BMD in addition to risk factors for fracture, such as long-term glucocorticoid therapy or hyperparathyroidism.

The NOF guidelines [11] for osteoporosis screening are among the most comprehensive and may have the most utility in clinical practice (Table 1.2) [11–19]. The NOF guidelines recommend screening for (1) women ≥65 years of age; (2) men ≥70 years of age; and (3) men and postmenopausal women ≥50 years of age with at least one risk factor for fracture. Risk factors include previous fracture, long-term glucocorticoid therapy, low body weight, family history of hip fracture, cigarette smoking, and excess alcohol intake.

Other guidelines are presented in Table 1.2. There is general consensus for screening women 65 years and older. Unfortunately, only up to 60% of women who qualify for bone density testing actually receive one [20]. The guidelines vary regarding recommendations for screening for younger women and men, with many not routinely recommending screening of men. Of concern is that up to 30% of osteoporotic fractures occur in men and male osteoporosis remains an underdiagnosed and undertreated condition [21]. In addition, the American College of Rheumatology guidelines recommend screening patients starting glucocorticoid therapy with plan for prednisone at >2.5 mg/day for ≥3 months [22]. International guidelines also recommend screening women starting aromatase inhibitor therapy or other endocrine treatments associated with bone loss [23].

In 2008, the University of Sheffield together with the WHO launched a Fracture Risk Assessment Tool (FRAX) [24]. FRAX is a fracture risk calculator that generates estimates of the 10-year absolute risk of major osteoporotic fractures and hip fractures. The calculator uses clinical risk factors that have been demonstrated to contribute to fracture risk independent of bone density. Fracture risk can be calculated with or without the input of BMD at the femoral neck by DXA. FRAX generates country-specific fracture risk, with different countries having different criteria for treatment; in the United States, the cutoffs are ≥20% for major

Table 1.2 Guidelines for osteoporosis screening

American College of Obstetrics and Gynecology (ACOG)	The ACOG [13] recommends measurement of BMD (DXA) in:
	   Women ≥65 years
	   Postmenopausal women <65 years with one or more risk factors for osteoporosis
	   Postmenopausal women with a history of fracture

American College of Preventative Medicine (ACPM)	The ACPM [14] recommends measurement of BMD (DXA) in:
	   Women ≥65 years
	   Men ≥70 years
	   Younger postmenopausal women and men 50–69 years with additional clinical risk factors for fracture

Association of Clinical Endocrinologists (AACE)	AACE [15] recommends measurement of BMD (DXA of the hip and spine) in:
	   Women ≥65 years
	   Postmenopausal women with a history of fracture
	   Postmenopausal women with osteopenia identified radiographically
	   Postmenopausal women starting or taking glucocorticoid therapy ≥3 months
	   Other perimenopausal or postmenopausal women with risk factors for osteoporosis if willing to consider pharmacologic therapy
	   Patients with secondary osteoporosis
	Vertebral imaging is recommended when T-score is <−1.0 if any of the following are present:
	   Women ≥70 years
	   Men ≥80 years
	   Historical height loss of >4 cm (>1.5 inches)
	   Self-reported but undocumented history of vertebral fracture
	   Glucocorticoid therapy ≥5 mg of prednisone or equivalent for ≥3 months

Endocrine Society (ES)	ES [16] recommends measurement of BMD (DXA of the hip and spine) in:
	   Men ≥70 years
	   Men ≥50 years with risk factors for fracture
	   Men ≥50 years with a history of fracture
	   No formal recommendations given for women
	The 33% forearm (one-third radius) site is recommended in the following cases:
	   If hip and/or spine cannot be measured or interpreted
	   Hyperparathyroidism
	   Men receiving androgen deprivation therapy for prostate cancer

(continued)

Table 1.2 (continued)

International Society for Clinical Densitometry (ISCD)	The ISCD [12] recommends measurement of BMD (DXA of the hip and spine) in:
	  Women ≥65 years
	  Men ≥70 years
	  Postmenopausal women <65 years and men <70 years with risk factors for fracture
	  Women during the menopausal transition with risk factors for fracture
	  Adults with a fragility fracture
	  Adults with a disease or condition associated with low bone mass or bone loss
	  Anyone being considered for pharmacologic therapy for osteoporosis
	  Anyone not receiving therapy when evidence of bone loss would lead to treatment
	  Postmenopausal women discontinuing estrogen
	The 33% forearm (one-third radius) site is recommended in the following cases:
	  If hip and/or spine cannot be measured or interpreted
	  Hyperparathyroidism
	  Severe obesity (over the weight limit of DXA table)
	Vertebral fracture assessment is recommended when T-score is <−1.0 if any of the following are present:
	  Women ≥70 years
	  Men ≥80 years
	  Historical height loss of >4 cm (>1.5 inches)
	  Self-reported but undocumented history of vertebral fracture
	  Glucocorticoid therapy ≥5 mg of prednisone or equivalent for ≥3 months

National Osteoporosis Foundation (NOF)	The NOF [11] recommends measurement of BMD (DXA of the hip and spine) in:
	  Women ≥65 years
	  Men ≥70 years
	  Postmenopausal women <65 years and men <70 years with risk factors for fracture
	  Adults with a fragility fracture
	Vertebral imaging is recommended if any of the following are present:
	  Women ≥70 years and men ≥80 years with T-score ≤−1.0
	  Women 65–69 years and men 70–79 years with T-score ≤−1.5
	  Postmenopausal women and men ≥50 years if risk factors are present

Table 1.2 (continued)

North American Menopause Society (NAMS)	The NAMS [17] recommends measurement of BMD (DXA) in:
	  Women ≥65 years
	  Postmenopausal women ≥50 years with risk factors

United States Preventative Services Task Force (USPSTF)	The USPSTF [18] recommends measurement of BMD (DXA) in:
	  Postmenopausal women ≥65 years
	  Postmenopausal women <65 years with FRAX 10-year risk of major osteoporotic fracture of ≥8.4%

UK National Osteoporosis Guideline Group (NOGG)	The NOGG [19] recommends:
	  Fracture probability assessment using FRAX in postmenopausal women and men ≥50 who have risk factors for fracture. In individuals at intermediate risk, BMD measurements should be performed using DXA and fracture probability re-estimated using FRAX
	  Vertebral fracture assessment in postmenopausal women and men age >50 years if there is a history of ≥4 cm height loss, kyphosis, recent or current long-term oral glucocorticoid therapy, or a BMD T-score ≤−2.5

osteoporotic fractures and ≥3.0% for hip fractures. The American Association of Clinical Endocrinology and National Bone Health Alliance Working Group recommend that a diagnosis of osteoporosis be made in the setting of elevated fracture risk calculated by FRAX [15, 25].

Identification of a previously undetected vertebral fracture can change the diagnostic classification of a patient (as in the case presented above) and may guide the choice of initial therapy. Vertebral fractures are a strong predictor of future fractures of all types. While they are the most common fragility fracture, up to 75% of vertebral fractures do not present with clinical symptoms, and vertebral fractures are significantly underdiagnosed [26]. Vertebral fracture assessment (VFA) is a method of visualizing spine fractures using the DXA machine at the time of BMD testing. VFA can detect moderate-to-severe vertebral fractures similarly to radiographs but with much less radiation exposure and lower cost. In one study of postmenopausal women 65 years and older, the sensitivity and specificity of VFA for severe and moderate fractures were 87–93% and 93–95%, respectively. VFA performs less well for detection of mild fractures [27]. The ISCD guidelines recommend VFA for patients when T-score is <-1.0 if any one or more of the following are present: (1) women ≥ 70 years or men ≥ 80 years; (2) historical height loss of >4 cm (>1.5 inches); (3) self-reported but undocumented history of vertebral fracture; and (4) glucocorticoid therapy ≥ 5 mg of prednisone or equivalent for ≥ 3 months [12, 15]. The NOF, American Association of Clinical Endocrinology, and Endocrine Society guidelines recommend vertebral imaging as per Table 1.2. Guidelines from the Fourth International Workshop on the Management of Asymptomatic Primary Hyperparathyroidism also recommend vertebral imaging to exclude fracture in patients with asymptomatic primary hyperparathyroidism [28].

Peripheral DXA and quantitative ultrasonagraphy have been used for screening but are not standardized for use with the WHO classification system, other than distal radius measurement by peripheral DXA. Quantitative computed tomography (CT) and high-resolution peripheral quantitative CT can measure volumetric BMD but are primarily used in research studies and not widely clinically available [29].

Bone turnover markers have been demonstrated in some studies, but not all, to predict fracture risk independent of BMD, with insufficient data for their use in fracture risk stratification in clinical practice [30].

Management

Most osteoporotic fractures occur in patients with osteopenia by bone density classification, not osteoporosis [31]. This is in part because there are many more patients in this category. Patients with normal bone density can also sustain a fragility fracture with subsequent diagnosis of osteoporosis, however. Bone strength, which determines fracture risk, reflects the integration of bone density, which is easily measured by DXA, as well as bone quality, which is not measured by DXA [32]. Bone quality includes the macro- and microstructural characteristics of bone tissue, easily characterized by bone biopsy or high-resolution technologies that are not routinely used. The clinical risk factors used in the FRAX tool are thought to contribute to bone quality [24]. In addition, trabecular bone score can provide a measurement of bone quality from the lumbar spine DXA image using proprietary software [33]. Chapter 3 further addresses FRAX, trabecular bone score, as well as other methods to calculate fracture risk.

The NOF guidelines recommend therapy for patients with a clinical diagnosis of osteoporosis by low-trauma hip or vertebral (clinical or morphometric) fracture, regardless of bone density measurement [11]. Treatment is recommended in patients with a DXA diagnosis of osteoporosis with T-score ≤ -2.5 at the lumbar spine or femoral neck after appropriate evaluation to exclude secondary causes. Patients with osteopenia and elevated fracture risk as calculated by FRAX should also be treated; in the United States, the cutoffs are $\geq 20\%$ for major osteoporotic fractures and $\geq 3.0\%$ for hip fractures [24].

Outcome

The patient was transitioned from hydroxychloroquine and prednisone to upadacitinib by his rheumatologist. His hyperparathyroidism resolved with calcium and vitamin D supplementation. The patient declined osteoanabolic therapy and was most amenable to treatment with zoledronic acid. His bone density demonstrated significant improvements at the spine and hip sites after two infusions. He has been able to remain off prednisone for the past 2 years. He has not sustained any fractures during therapy. The plan is to treat with zoledronic acid 5 mg IV annually for up to 6 years due to the HORIZON-PFT extension trial demonstrating benefit for morphometric vertebral fractures with up to 6 years of annual therapy [34].

Clinical Pearls/Pitfalls

- A diagnosis of osteoporosis can be made in the setting of a fragility fracture, defined as a fracture occurring from a force equivalent to a fall from standing height or less.
- It is preferable to make a diagnosis of osteoporosis in a patient prior to the occurrence of fracture through bone density testing using dual-energy X-ray absorptiometry (DXA).
- The National Osteoporosis Foundation guidelines recommend DXA screening for (1) women ≥65 years of age; (2) men ≥70 years of age; and (3) men and post-menopausal women ≥50 years of age with at least one risk factor for fracture. Risk factors include previous fracture, long-term glucocorticoid therapy, low body weight, family history of hip fracture, cigarette smoking, and excess alcohol intake.
- Identification of a previously undetected vertebral fracture can change the diagnosis of a patient to osteoporosis.
- The International Society for Clinical Densitometry recommends screening for vertebral fractures in patients with a T-score ≤1.0 if any one or more of the following are present: (1) women ≥70 years or men ≥80 years; (2) historical height loss of >4 cm (>1.5 inches); (3) self-reported but undocumented history of vertebral fracture; and (4) glucocorticoid therapy ≥5 mg of prednisone or equivalent for ≥3 months.

References

1. NIH Consensus Development Panel on Osteoporosis Prevention, Diagnosis, and Therapy. Osteoporosis prevention, diagnosis, and therapy. JAMA. 2001;285(6):785.
2. Wright NC, Looker AC, Saag KG, Curtis JR, Delzell ES, Randall S, Dawson-Hughes B. The recent prevalence of osteoporosis and low bone

mass in the United States based on bone mineral density at the femoral neck or lumbar spine. J Bone Miner Res. 2014;29(11):2520.

3. Burge R, Dawson-Hughes B, Solomon DH, Wong JB, King A, Tosteson A. Incidence and economic burden of osteoporosis-related fractures in the United States, 2005–2025. J Bone Miner Res. 2007;22(3):465.

4. Johnell O, Kanis JA. An estimate of the worldwide prevalence of disability associated with osteoporotic fractures. Osteoporos Int. 2006;17:1726.

5. Cummings SR, Black DM, Rubin SM. Lifetime risks of hip, Colles', or vertebral fracture and coronary heart disease among white postmenopausal women. Arch Intern Med. 1989;149:2445.

6. World Health Organization. WHO technical report series. Assessment of fracture risk and its application to screening for postmenopausal osteoporosis. Report of a WHO Study Group, vol. 843; 1994. p. 1–129.

7. Mundi S, Pindiprolu B, Simunovic N, Bhandari M. Similar mortality rates in hip fracture patients over the past 31 years. Acta Orthop. 2014;85(1):54–9.

8. Magaziner J, Hawkes W, Hebel JR, Zimmerman SI, Fox KM, Dolan M, Felsenthal G, Kenzora J. Recovery from hip fracture in eight areas of function. J Gerontol A Biol Sci Med Sci. 2000;55(9):M498–507.

9. Blake GM, Fogelman I. Technical principles of dual energy x-ray absorptiometry. Semin Nucl Med. 1997;27(3):210–28.

10. Blausen.com Staff. Medical gallery of Blausen Medical 2014. WikiJ Med. 2014;1(2) https://doi.org/10.15347/wjm/2014.010. ISSN 2002-4436. Own work.

11. Cosman F, de Beur SJ, LeBoff MS, Lewiecki EM, Tanner B, et al. Clinician's guide to prevention and treatment of osteoporosis. Osteoporos Int. 2014;25(10):2359–81.

12. Lewiecki EM, Watts NB, McClung MR, Petak SM, Bachrach LK, et al. Official positions of the international society for clinical densitometry. J Clin Endocrinol Metab. 2004;89:3651–5.

13. Committee on Practice Bulletins-Gynecology, The American College of Obstetricians and Gynecologists. ACOG Practice Bulletin N. 129. Osteoporosis. Obstet Gynecol. 2012;120(3):718–34.

14. Lim LS, Hoeksema LJ, Sherin K, ACPM Prevention Practice Committee. Screening for osteoporosis in the adult U.S. population: ACPM position statement on preventive practice. Am J Prev Med. 2009;36(4):366–75.

15. Camacho PM, Petak SM, Binkley N, Diab DL, Eldeiry LS, et al. American Association of Clinical Endocrinologists/American College of Endocrinology Clinical Practice Guidelines for the diagnosis and treatment of postmenopausal osteoporosis-2020 update. Endocr Pract. 2020;26(Suppl 1):1–46.

16. Watts NB, Adler RA, Bilezikian JP, Drake MT, Eastell R, et al. Osteoporosis in men: an Endocrine Society clinical practice guideline. J Clin Endocrinol Metab. 2012;97(6):1802–22.

17. North American Menopause Society. Management of osteoporosis in postmenopausal women: 2010 position statement of the North American Menopause Society. Menopause. 2010;17(1):25–54.
18. U.S. Preventive Services Task Force. Screening for osteoporosis in post-menopausal women: recommendations and rationale. Ann Intern Med. 2002;137:526–8.
19. Compston J, Cooper A, Cooper C, Gittoes N, Gregson C, et al. UK clinical guideline for the prevention and treatment of osteoporosis. Arch Osteoporos. 2017;12(1):43.
20. Alswat KA. Gender disparities in osteoporosis. J Clin Med Res. 2017;9(5):382–7.
21. Nelson T, Nelson SD, Newbold J, Nelson RE, LaFleur J. The clinical epidemiology of male osteoporosis: a review of the recent literature. Clin Epidemiol. 2015;7:65–76.
22. Buckley L, Guyatt G, Fink HA, Cannon M, Grossman J, et al. 2017 American College of Rheumatology Guideline for the prevention and treatment of glucocorticoid-induced osteoporosis. Arthritis Rheumatol. 2017;69(8):1521–37.
23. Hadji P, Aapro MS, Body JJ, Gnant M, Brandi ML, et al. Management of Aromatase Inhibitor-Associated Bone Loss (AIBL) in postmenopausal women with hormone sensitive breast cancer: joint position statement of the IOF, CABS, ECTS, IEG, ESCEO IMS, and SIOG. J Bone Oncol. 2017;7:1–12.
24. https://www.sheffield.ac.uk/FRAX/. Accessed 6/01/2021.
25. Siris ES, Adler R, Bilezikian J, Bolognese M, Dawson-Hughes B, Favus MJ, Harris ST, Jan de Beur SM, Khosla S, Lane NE, Lindsay R, Nana AD, Orwoll ES, Saag K, Silverman S, Watts NB. The clinical diagnosis of osteoporosis: a position statement from the National Bone Health Alliance Working Group. Osteoporos Int. 2014;25(5):1439–43.
26. Delmas PD, van de Largerjit L, Watts NB, Eastell R, Genant H, et al. Underdiagnosis of vertebral fractures is a worldwide problem: the IMPACT study. J Bone Miner Res. 2005;20:557–63.
27. Schousboe JT, Debold CR. Reliability and accuracy of vertebral fracture assessment with densitometry compared to radiography in clinical practice. Osteoporos Int. 2006;17(2):281–9.
28. Bilezikian JP, Brandi ML, Eastell R, Silverberg SJ, Udelsman R, et al. Guidelines for the management of asymptomatic primary hyperparathyroidism: summary statement from the Fourth International Workshop. J Clin Endocrinol Metab. 2014;99(10):3561–9.
29. Raisz LG. Clinical practice. Screening for osteoporosis. N Engl J Med. 2005;353:164.
30. Eastell R, Pigott T, Gossiel F, Naylor KE, Walsh JS, et al. DIAGNOSIS OF ENDOCRINE DISEASE: bone turnover markers: are they clinically useful? Eur J Endocrinol. 2018;178(1):R19–31.

31. Siris ES, Chen YT, Abbott TA, Barrett-Connor E, Miller PD, et al. Bone mineral density thresholds for pharmacological intervention to prevent fractures. Arch Intern Med. 2004;164(10):1108–12.
32. Watts NB. Bone quality: getting closer to a definition. J Bone Miner Res. 2002;17(7):1148–50.
33. Silva BC, Leslie WD, Resch H, Lamy O, Lesnyak O, et al. Trabecular bone score: a noninvasive analytical method based upon the DXA image. J Bone Miner Res. 2014;29(3):518–30.
34. Black DM, Reid IR, Boonen S, Bucci-Rectweg C, Cauley JA, et al. The effect of 3 versus 6 years of zoledronic acid treatment of osteoporosis: a randomized extension to the HORIZON-Pivotal Fracture Trial (PFT). J Bone Miner Res. 2012;27(2):243–54.

Nutrition and Lifestyle Approaches to Optimize Skeletal Health

2

Joanne Bruno and Melissa Sum

Case Presentation

A 68-year-old woman with no significant past medical history is found to have osteopenia on a bone density screening.

She had no personal or family history of bone fractures. Menstrual history was notable for menarche at age 13, regular menses, menopause at age 52, and no children. She took cholecalciferol 1000 IU daily. Her dietary calcium included one serving of calcium-rich food per week. She exercised 6 days/week, which consisted of a combination of walking, yoga, and Pilates.

Her physical exam was unremarkable. Laboratory evaluation for secondary causes of osteopenia showed normal comprehensive metabolic panel, thyroid function testing, and parathyroid hormone levels. Her 25-hydroxyvitamin D level was 30.2 ng/mL. The patient's recent bone density scan was significant for the following T-scores: lumbar spine −1.6, femoral neck −1.3, and total hip −0.9 with significant declines in the spine and total hip compared to 2 years ago. Her FRAX score estimated 10-year risks of major

J. Bruno · M. Sum (✉)
Division of Endocrinology, Diabetes, and Metabolism,
Department of Medicine, New York University Langone Medical Center,
New York, NY, USA
e-mail: Melissa.Sum@nyulangone.org

© The Author(s), under exclusive license to Springer Nature
Switzerland AG 2021
N. E. Cusano (ed.), *Osteoporosis*,
https://doi.org/10.1007/978-3-030-83951-2_2

osteoporotic fracture and hip fracture to be 9.3% and 1.1%, respectively, not meeting criteria for pharmacologic treatment.

The patient inquired about lifestyle changes to optimize her bone health.

Management

Nutrition

Calcium and vitamin D are the most prominent supplements studied with regard to bone health. In healthy bone, bone formation and resorption occur in concert without significant net change in bone mass. Dysregulation of calcium and vitamin D metabolism impacts these pathways and can result in bone pathology. Other essential nutrients such as vitamin K and strontium have also been investigated for their role in bone metabolism. This section reviews the data involving these nutrients and bone health (Table 2.1).

As an essential element, calcium enters the body solely through dietary means and is incorporated into bone as calcium hydroxyapatite, which enhances bone strength. Calcium absorption in the gut and excretion via both intestinal and renal mechanisms are regulated via a hormonal system that utilizes parathyroid hormone, calcitriol, ionized calcium, and the calcium-sensing receptor (CaSR) to maintain calcium homeostasis [4]. The most common cause of absorptive hypocalcemia is vitamin D deficiency, as vitamin D is essential for facilitating intestinal calcium uptake [5]. Both chronic hypocalcemia and chronic vitamin D deficiency result in persistently elevated parathyroid hormone levels, causing excessive bone resorption and ultimately bone loss if untreated [6].

While it is undisputed that calcium and vitamin D deficiency, especially during adolescence, result in bone pathology, their role in postmenopausal osteoporosis is less clear [7]. To date, most professional organizations have based their guidelines for optimal calcium intake on calcium balance studies, which explore the amount of calcium intake required to achieve neutral calcium

Table 2.1 Summary of nutrients with a role or possible role in bone health

	Recommended daily dose	Dietary sources	Risks
Calcium	1200 mg [1]	Dairy products (milk, cheese, yogurt) Green leafy vegetables (kale, okra, spinach) Calcium-fortified beverages (almond milk, soy milk, juices) Dried peas and beans Fish with bones	Increased risk of renal calculi with supplemental doses greater than 1200 mg daily [1]
Vitamin D	1000 IU daily, titrated to achieve goal level 20–30 ng/mL [1]	Oily fish (salmon, sardines, herring, mackerel) Red meat Liver Egg yolks Vitamin D-fortified foods (dairy, breakfast cereals)	Can increase risk for high calcium levels if excessive intake
Vitamin K	90 mcg/day [2]	Leafy greens Carrots Tomatoes Legumes and peas Red meat Tuna Natto Cheese	
Strontium	No specific recommended dose, tested in clinical trials at doses of 2 g daily	Seafood Seaweed	Supplementation associated with increased risk of venous thromboembolism, pulmonary embolism, and myocardial infarction [3]

balance [8]. One recent study reports that calcium balance can be maintained across a wide range of dietary calcium intake: 415–1740 mg/day [9], which suggests a robust internal mechanism for maintaining calcium homeostasis and calls into question the role of supplementation if an individual's dietary intake falls within this range [9]. The relationship between calcium balance and bone density or fracture risk has not been proven; thus, the clinical implications of these studies have yet to be determined.

Despite this, establishing the effect of calcium and vitamin D on bone health carries great clinical significance. A number of prospective cohort studies designed to investigate the impact of calcium intake on bone loss have been completed, with the majority showing no relationship between the two at any site [7]. The United States Preventive Services Task Force (USPSTF) 2018 guidelines reviewed 8 randomized clinical trials examining the effects of vitamin D, calcium, or combined supplementation on primary prevention of fractures in postmenopausal women without a known disorder related to bone metabolism [10]. Of the four studies that examined the role of vitamin D supplementation alone, two evaluated daily doses of 400 IU or less and two evaluated higher dose supplementation [10]. One of the studies using high-dose vitamin D supplementation found a significant reduction in total fractures, while the others showed no significant difference [10]. Two studies that examined the role of calcium supplementation found no significant differences in fracture outcomes, though these studies were not adequately powered to detect differences [10]. The combined vitamin D/calcium supplementation trials also had mixed results, with the larger Women's Health Initiative trial finding no statistically significant difference in fracture risk and a smaller trial finding a significant reduction in nonvertebral fractures with vitamin D and calcium supplementation [10]. Given the lack of overwhelming positive data to support calcium and vitamin D supplementation in the general population, the USPSTF recommends against routine calcium and vitamin D supplementation in those without specific indications [10].

In contrast, supplementation for individuals with metabolic bone diseases such as osteoporosis or vitamin D deficiency is beneficial. In a meta-analysis of 107 randomized controlled trials examining the efficacy of various pharmacological therapies for postmenopausal women with primary osteoporosis, combined calcium and vitamin D supplementation significantly reduced the risk of hip fracture (RR 0.81) compared to placebo [6]. Calcium supplementation alone had no significant effect on fracture risk [6]. The doses of calcium and vitamin D used in these trials varied significantly, ranging from 400 to 300,000 IU of vitamin D daily and 1–1.2 g of calcium daily, so the optimal dose range remains unclear [6]. Similarly, the DIPART study, a meta-analysis of seven major randomized trials that looked at the effects of vitamin D supplementation, either alone or combined with calcium, found that trials using vitamin D (400–800 IU daily) with calcium (1 g daily) showed a reduced risk of overall fracture (HR 0.92) and hip fracture (HR 0.84), whereas using vitamin D alone at doses of either 400 or 800 IU daily had no significant effects on fracture risk [11]. One theory is that that combination therapy more effectively treats secondary hyperparathyroidism. Nearly all recent trials involving pharmacological therapies for osteoporosis use calcium and vitamin D supplementation in their study design, and so the antifracture efficacy of these medications is predicated on the concurrent use of these supplements [1]. Thus, any treatment regimen for osteoporosis should include adequate intake of calcium and vitamin D to simulate trial conditions.

Endocrine Society recommends a daily calcium intake of 1200 mg/day for postmenopausal women with osteoporosis, including both supplemental and dietary calcium, with preference for dietary intake [1]. This daily calcium intake should be consumed in smaller doses throughout the day as absorption can decline as the amount of elemental calcium consumed at once increases, with optimal absorption at doses ≤500 mg [8]. Supplemental calcium use upward of 1000 mg/day has been linked to increased risk of renal calculi [1]. There has also been recent speculation as to whether calcium supplementation is associated with increased risk of cardiovascular disease [1]. The largest study to date exploring this is the Women's Health Initiative, which randomized 36,282 healthy postmenopausal women to receive either calcium carbonate 500 mg with vitamin D 200 IU twice per day or placebo and found no differences with regard to incidence of myocardial infarction, coronary heart disease death, or stroke [12]. However, approximately 50% of participants in this study were taking personal (non-protocol) calcium and vitamin D supplements at randomization and were allowed to continue the use of these supplements in addition to study medications, potentially obscuring any positive results [13]. When the data was reanalyzed to exclude women who were taking calcium supplements prior to randomization, a positive interaction was found between calcium/vitamin D supplementation, myocardial infarction (HR 1.22, $P = 0.05$), and stroke (HR 1.16, $P = 0.05$) [13]. However, when daily supplement intake was stratified according to reported dose, no dose relationship was found between any of these endpoints [13]. Additionally, no relationship was found between increased dietary intake of calcium and incidence of cardiovascular disease [13]. Given that association does not prove causation, additional research is needed to investigate whether there might be a causative relationship between calcium supplementation and cardiovascular disease. Until those data are available, discretion should be used regarding recommendation of calcium supplementation, with a preference toward recommending dietary calcium. In postmenopausal women with low bone mineral density and at high risk of fracture with osteoporosis, vitamin D supplementation should be titrated to achieve a goal 25-hydroxyvitamin D level of at least 30 ng/mL per Endocrine Society guidelines or 20 ng/mL per European guidelines, with a dose of 1000 IU daily usually being sufficient to meet these targets [1, 14]. Vitamin D-rich foods include oily fish, red meat, liver, and egg yolks, as well as other fortified foods.

Vitamin K is another essential nutrient that has been implicated in bone health. It naturally occurs in a wide variety of foods including leafy greens, carrots, tomatoes, legumes, peas, red meat, and tuna. In addition to its established role in blood coagulation, it is thought to also be important for promoting osteoblast-to-osteocyte transition and for limiting osteoclastogenesis through its action as a cofactor for carboxylation of bone matrix proteins [15]. Newer data also suggest a role for vitamin K in regulating the transcription programs underlying osteoblastogenesis and osteoclastogenesis [16]. A subset of studies have shown a positive effect of vitamin K supplementation on BMD at doses of 100 mcg/day in healthy postmenopausal women, specifically at the lumbar spine [17]. However, others have also shown no effect of vitamin K supplementation on bone mineral density at higher supplement doses [15]. Data on the efficacy of vitamin K supplementation in lowering fracture risk is similarly mixed. A meta-analysis of seven trials investigating the relationship between fractures and vitamin K showed that vitamin K supplementation appeared to reduce hip (OR 0.23, 95% CI, 0.12–0.47), vertebral (OR 0.40; 95% CI, 0.25–0.65), and nonvertebral fracture risk (OR 0.19; 95% CI, 0.11–0.35), though most of these positive effects were attributed to just one of the included studies [18], whereas multiple other studies have shown no effect of vitamin K supplementation on fracture risk [15]. The majority of studies investigating vitamin K supplementation were completed in Asia, and in Japan it has been approved for use in the prevention and treatment of osteoporosis [19]. Few studies were performed in other populations. Given variability in study design, vitamin K formulation and dosage, and study population selection, it is difficult to draw any strong conclusions on vitamin K usage for bone health.

Strontium ranelate is a trace element found in seawater and soil. It is chemically similar to calcium and can mimic calcium's physiologic actions including binding to the calcium-sensing receptor on osteoblasts and osteoclasts, promoting osteoblast formation and activity, and inhibiting osteoclast activity and survival [20]. Two major phase III clinical trials have examined the role of strontium ranelate supplementation in postmenopausal women with osteoporosis. One investigated the effects of strontium ranelate treatment on the risk of vertebral fractures, and the other examined its effects on nonvertebral fractures [21, 22]. Both studies utilized a strontium ranelate dose of 2 g/day and followed study participants over 3 years. The first study found that treatment with strontium ranelate resulted in a decrease in new vertebral fractures (RR 0.59, 95% CI 0.48–0.73) as well as a statistically significant increase in bone mineral density in both the lumbar spine and the femoral neck (14.4% and 8.3%, respectively) [21]. The second study found that treatment with strontium ranelate resulted in relative risk reduction of nonvertebral fractures by

16% and reduction in major fragility fractures by 19%; it also significantly increased bone mineral density at the femoral neck and total hip (8.2% and 9.8%, respectively) [22]. Both studies reported a similar incidence in adverse events between the treatment and placebo groups. While it is not currently approved for use in the United States, strontium ranelate is used as a prescription drug in other areas of the world for treatment of postmenopausal osteoporosis. However, it has been associated with increased risk of venous thromboembolism, pulmonary embolism, and myocardial infarction, and in countries where it is approved, its use is now restricted to those with severe osteoporosis without other treatment options [3].

Lifestyle

Modifiable lifestyle factors such as exercise and physical activity have also been shown to affect adult peak bone mass via a positive effect of mechanical loads on osteogenesis [23]. A systematic review of prospective cohort studies found positive associations between physical activity and BMD, especially at weight-bearing sites [23]. Additionally, more frequent positive associations were seen when physical activity was maintained from adolescence through adulthood than when it was isolated, indicating the importance of consistency over an individual's lifespan [23].

Additional questions regarding exercise type and frequency to optimize bone health remain [23, 24]. This is in part due to high levels of heterogeneity among studies. Based on the above data, it makes sense that exercise programs aiming to improve bone health should target load-bearing regions of the skeleton, including weight-lifting exercises such as leg presses, leg extensions, leg curls, and squats as well as high-impact exercises such as jumping, running, and stair climbing [25] (Fig. 2.1). Specific exercise regimens must accommodate an individual patient's fall risk and exercise tolerance [25]. At least 2–3 days of exercise per week for at least 30–60 minutes per session are recommended, or as much as can be tolerated [25]. Dynamic loading exercises of short load duration that are nonrepetitive in load direction (i.e., tennis, high-intensity interval training, jumping, tumbling) may

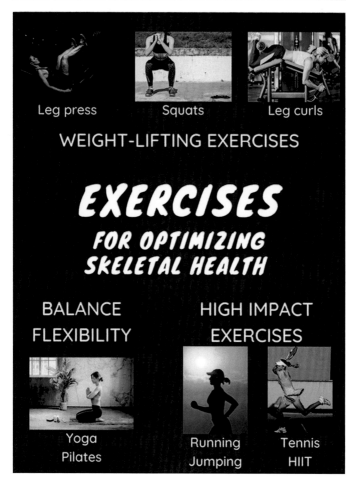

Fig. 2.1 An exercise regimen consisting of a combination of strength training, high-impact activities, and flexibility training is beneficial for bone health and fracture prevention. (Images used per Canva.com's Free Media License Agreement)

be more effective than static loading exercises with repetitive motions of longer duration [25, 26] (Fig. 2.1). Additionally, exercise regimens that enhance balance and flexibility such as yoga, Pilates, and Tai Chi are thought to help in fall prevention [26]

(Fig. 2.1). While these interventions have the highest impact when implemented during childhood and adolescence, they likely have some beneficial effects even in elderly adults [26].

Other modifiable risk factors for optimizing bone health include abstaining from cigarette smoking and limiting alcohol use, as the former has been clearly associated with decreased bone density and the latter increases risk of falls [24]. Thus, all patients should undergo screening for substance use and appropriate counseling if indicated.

Outcome

The patient was counseled to increase intake of calcium-rich foods in order to meet the recommended daily dose of 1200 mg calcium/day for those with metabolic bone disease. If she were to be unable to meet the goal from dietary intake, calcium supplementation would be considered. She continued her daily vitamin D supplement. She was also instructed to add high-intensity interval training into her exercise regimen, if possible, and to discuss her progress in 6 months with a plan to repeat bone density measurement in 2 years.

Over the subsequent 6 months, the patient was able to increase her calcium intake to three servings of calcium-rich foods per day (8 oz milk, 6 oz yogurt, 1.5 oz cheese). She also started a home exercise program that included a combination of high-intensity interval training, yoga, Pilates, and weight lifting. Her bone density will be repeated in 18 months.

Clinical Pearls/Pitfalls
- Calcium and vitamin D play a critical role in bone development and homeostasis with sufficient intake being critical during adolescence for maintaining normal bone physiology. However, in healthy adults, supplementation

with calcium and/or vitamin D has not been shown to have a positive effect on bone health and is not routinely recommended.

- In patients with underlying metabolic bone disease, combined calcium and vitamin D supplementation is recommended to achieve daily calcium intake of 1200 mg/day (in divided doses) and 25-hydroxy vitamin D levels of 20–30 ng/mL. Calcium intake should occur primarily through dietary means as supplemental calcium pills have been associated with an increased risk of renal calculi and possibly increased cardiovascular risk.
- Vitamin K and strontium ranelate are posited to have a positive effect on bone health and are approved for use in treatment of osteoporosis in various parts of the world; however, more studies are needed to further clarify their effectiveness, risks, and optimal dosage.
- Physical activity has a positive effect on bone structure with the greatest benefits seen on load-bearing joints and when exercise is sustained over the lifespan. A combination of strength training, high-impact activities, and exercises that emphasize flexibility and/or balance have all been shown to be beneficial for bone health and fracture prevention.

References

1. Eastell R, et al. Pharmacological management of osteoporosis in postmenopausal women: an Endocrine Society* clinical practice guideline. J Clin Endocrinol Metab. 2019;104(5):1595–622.
2. Trumbo P, et al. Dietary reference intakes: vitamin A, vitamin K, arsenic, boron, chromium, copper, iodine, iron, manganese, molybdenum, nickel, silicon, vanadium, and zinc. J Am Diet Assoc. 2001;101(3):294–301.
3. Reginster JY. Cardiac concerns associated with strontium ranelate. Expert Opin Drug Saf. 2014;13(9):1209–13.

4. Peacock M. Calcium metabolism in health and disease. Clin J Am Soc Nephrol. 2010;5(Suppl 1):S23–30.

5. Lips P, van Schoor NM. The effect of vitamin D on bone and osteoporosis. Best Pract Res Clin Endocrinol Metab. 2011;25(4):585–91.

6. Barrionuevo P, et al. Efficacy of pharmacological therapies for the prevention of fractures in postmenopausal women: a network meta-analysis. J Clin Endocrinol Metab. 2019;104(5):1623–30.

7. Reid IR, Bristow SM, Bolland MJ. Calcium supplements: benefits and risks. J Intern Med. 2015;278(4):354–68.

8. Ross AC. The 2011 report on dietary reference intakes for calcium and vitamin D. Public Health Nutr. 2011;14(5):938–9.

9. Hunt CD, Johnson LK. Calcium requirements: new estimations for men and women by cross-sectional statistical analyses of calcium balance data from metabolic studies. Am J Clin Nutr. 2007;86(4):1054–63.

10. US Preventive Services Task Force, et al. Vitamin D, calcium, or combined supplementation for the primary prevention of fractures in community-dwelling adults: US Preventive Services Task Force recommendation statement. JAMA. 2018;319(15):1592–9.

11. DIPART Group. Patient level pooled analysis of 68 500 patients from seven major vitamin D fracture trials in US and Europe. BMJ. 2010;340:b5463.

12. Hsia J, et al. Calcium/vitamin D supplementation and cardiovascular events. Circulation. 2007;115(7):846–54.

13. Bolland MJ, et al. Calcium supplements with or without vitamin D and risk of cardiovascular events: reanalysis of the Women's Health Initiative limited access dataset and meta-analysis. BMJ. 2011;342:d2040.

14. Ebeling PR, et al. MANAGEMENT OF ENDOCRINE DISEASE: therapeutics of vitamin D. Eur J Endocrinol. 2018;179(5):R239–59.

15. Palermo A, et al. Vitamin K and osteoporosis: myth or reality? Metabolism. 2017;70:57–71.

16. Yamaguchi M, Weitzmann MN. Vitamin K2 stimulates osteoblastogenesis and suppresses osteoclastogenesis by suppressing NF-kappaB activation. Int J Mol Med. 2011;27(1):3–14.

17. Kanellakis S, et al. Changes in parameters of bone metabolism in postmenopausal women following a 12-month intervention period using dairy products enriched with calcium, vitamin D, and phylloquinone (vitamin K(1)) or menaquinone-7 (vitamin K (2)): the Postmenopausal Health Study II. Calcif Tissue Int. 2012;90(4):251–62.

18. Cockayne S, et al. Vitamin K and the prevention of fractures: systematic review and meta-analysis of randomized controlled trials. Arch Intern Med. 2006;166(12):1256–61.

19. Ishida Y. Vitamin K2. Clin Calcium. 2008;18(10):1476–82.

20. Fonseca JE, Brandi ML. Mechanism of action of strontium ranelate: what are the facts? Clin Cases Miner Bone Metab. 2010;7(1):17–8.

21. Meunier PJ, et al. The effects of strontium ranelate on the risk of vertebral fracture in women with postmenopausal osteoporosis. N Engl J Med. 2004;350(5):459–68.
22. Reginster JY, et al. Strontium ranelate reduces the risk of nonvertebral fractures in postmenopausal women with osteoporosis: Treatment of Peripheral Osteoporosis (TROPOS) study. J Clin Endocrinol Metab. 2005;90(5):2816–22.
23. Bielemann RM, Martinez-Mesa J, Gigante DP. Physical activity during life course and bone mass: a systematic review of methods and findings from cohort studies with young adults. BMC Musculoskelet Disord. 2013;14:77.
24. Black DM, Rosen CJ. Clinical practice. Postmenopausal osteoporosis. N Engl J Med. 2016;374(3):254–62.
25. Guadalupe-Grau A, et al. Exercise and bone mass in adults. Sports Med. 2009;39(6):439–68.
26. Turner CH, Robling AG. Designing exercise regimens to increase bone strength. Exerc Sport Sci Rev. 2003;31(1):45–50.

The Utility and Applicability of Risk Assessment Tools and Trabecular Bone Score

3

Barbara C. Silva [ID]
and Maria Marta Sarquis Soares

Case Presentation

A 51-year-old Brazilian perimenopausal woman presented to the emergency department with right wrist pain after a fall from standing height. Right wrist radiographs confirmed a distal radius fracture associated with ulnar styloid fracture, successfully treated by closed reduction and cast immobilization. Her stature was 172 cm, with a body weight of 71.4 kg, and a body mass index (BMI) of 24.1 kg/m². Her physical examination was otherwise unremarkable. Her medical history included hypertension, dyslipidemia, impaired glucose tolerance, and vitiligo. She was

B. C. Silva (✉)
Endocrinology Division, Felicio Rocho Hospital, Belo Horizonte, Brazil

Endocrinology Division, Santa Casa Hospital, Belo Horizonte, Brazil

Department of Medicine, Centro Universitario de Belo Horizonte (UNI-BH), Belo Horizonte, Brazil

M. M. S. Soares
Endocrinology Division, Felicio Rocho Hospital, Belo Horizonte, Brazil

Department of Medicine, Federal University of Minas Gerais (UFMG), Belo Horizonte, Brazil

© The Author(s), under exclusive license to Springer Nature
Switzerland AG 2021
N. E. Cusano (ed.), *Osteoporosis*,
https://doi.org/10.1007/978-3-030-83951-2_3

compliant with atenolol, hydrochlorothiazide, and simvastatin. Her family history was positive for type 2 diabetes, but negative for fractures. She denied smoking or alcohol consumption, and her diet was low in calcium. The patient's menopause occurred approximately 6 months after her first evaluation, at the age of 52, but she did not have significant hot flashes or other bothersome menopausal symptoms.

Initial workup revealed a bone mineral density by DXA in the osteopenic range, with a T-score of -2.3 at the lumbar spine, -2.3 at the femoral neck, and -2.1 at the total hip. Trabecular bone score (TBS) was low at 1.11. Secondary causes of osteoporosis were excluded based on extensive laboratory evaluation that included complete blood count, serum calcium, phosphate, total protein, albumin, liver enzymes, alkaline phosphatase, creatinine, 25-hydroxyvitamin D, intact parathyroid hormone, TSH, tissue transglutaminase antibodies, and urinary calcium. The bone resorption marker, serum C-terminal telopeptide (CTX), was 0.447 ng/mL (reference range for premenopausal women: 0.025–0.573 ng/mL). Spine radiographs did not show vertebral fractures.

The patient's 10-year fracture probability was calculated using the Fracture Risk Assessment Tool (FRAX) with BMD. The TBS-adjusted FRAX was also assessed. The risks of major osteoporotic fracture (MOF) and hip fracture were, respectively, 7.4% and 1.8%, and after adjusting for TBS, 12% and 3.7% (Fig. 3.1). The 10-year probability of MOF and hip fractures exceeded the country-specific intervention thresholds by 20%, using both FRAX and TBS-adjusted FRAX, which would identify this patient as having a very high risk of fracture. Thus, despite the BMD in the osteopenic range, pharmacologic therapy with alendronate was recommended based on her history of prior fragility fracture and the finding of a very high fracture risk by FRAX. She was also counseled to keep an active lifestyle, including weight-bearing exercises, to adopt fall prevention strategies, and to increase her intake of calcium to 1200 mg/day from diet and supplements. Vitamin D supplements were also indicated to maintain her serum level of 25-hydroxyvitamin D above 30 ng/mL.

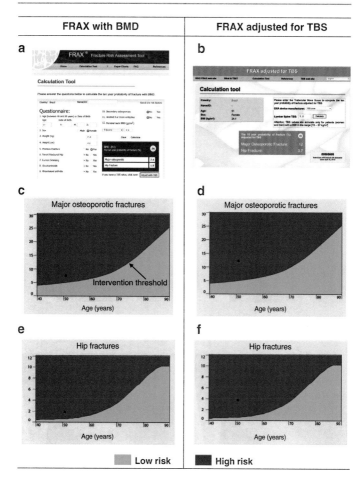

Fig. 3.1 Output of FRAX Brazil v4.2 (**a**), adjusted for TBS (**b**). Age-specific 10-year probability of major osteoporotic fracture (**c, d**) and hip fracture (**e, f**) for Brazilian women, as proposed by the UK National Osteoporosis Guideline Group (NOGG). The line denotes intervention thresholds for Brazilian women, which at the age of 51 years corresponds to 5% for major osteoporotic fractures and 0.7% for hip fractures. Dots represent, respectively, major osteoporotic and hip fracture probabilities of 7.4% (**c**) and 1.8% (**e**) using FRAX with BMD, and 12% (**d**) and 3.7% (**f**), using the TBS-adjusted FRAX. It is noted that the 10-year probabilities of fractures exceed the intervention thresholds by 20%, using both FRAX and TBS-adjusted FRAX. BMD, bone mineral density; BMI, body mass index; TBS, trabecular bone score; FRAX, Fracture Risk Assessment Tool

Assessment and Diagnosis

This patient experienced a typical osteoporotic fracture despite having a BMD by DXA in the osteopenic range. In fact, although low BMD is a strong predictor of fracture, most individuals with fragility fractures have BMD values that do not fall within the osteoporotic range [1, 2]. Thus, skeletal and extraskeletal risk factors that contribute to overall fracture risk should be identified to better select patients for treatment.

Among extraskeletal features, readily assessable clinical risk factors contribute to fracture risk, independently of BMD, and have been incorporated in risk assessment tools to calculate an individual's probability of fracture. FRAX is the most widely used and comprehensively evaluated risk assessment tool currently available [3]. It integrates the following risk factors: age, BMI, sex, previous fragility fracture, parental history of hip fracture, smoking, prolonged glucocorticoid use, rheumatoid arthritis, excessive alcohol consumption, and other causes of secondary osteoporosis. FRAX was developed through a series of meta-analyses of prospective cohort studies from Europe, North America, Asia, and Australia including more than 40,000 individuals. Its ability to predict fractures has been validated in independent cohorts [4–6]. FRAX incorporates the risk of fracture with risk of death, and country-specific FRAX calculators have been developed to account for geographical variations in fracture incidence and mortality [7]. The tool estimates 10-year probabilities of major osteoporotic fractures (clinical spine, hip, distal forearm, and proximal humerus) and hip fractures, in individuals between the ages of 40 and 90 years [7].

FRAX does not directly yield an indication for treatment [8]. The estimated FRAX-probability of fracture needs to be interpreted, and thresholds set above which pharmaceutical intervention is justified. To this end, the cost-effectiveness of a therapy can be considered to set the intervention threshold. Alternatively, the threshold can be clinically derived and then validated using a cost-effectiveness analysis [8]. The approach to set the threshold varies across the world. The National Osteoporosis Foundation in the United States recommends treatment for those with BMD in the osteopenic range associated with a 10-year FRAX-probability of major osteoporotic fractures ≥20% or hip fracture ≥3% from a cost-effectiveness analysis [9]. In contrast, the UK National Osteoporosis Guideline Group (NOGG) developed its guidance on the basis of clinical appropriateness, setting the threshold at the age-specific 10-year FRAX-probability of fracture equivalent to women having already sustained a fracture. This approach has also been shown to be cost-effective, being adopted in many countries, particularly in Europe and Latin America [7, 8].

The probability of fracture can be estimated with or without femoral neck BMD [7]. When the assessment is made without BMD, fracture probability will be categorized as low, intermediate, or high. Patients with intermediate risk of fracture should undergo a DXA test, whereas patients with high fracture risk should be considered for treatment. When the assessment is made with BMD, two categories will be defined, namely, low and high fracture risk. Recently, the International Osteoporosis Foundation (IOF) and the European Society for Clinical and Economic Evaluation of Osteoporosis and Osteoarthritis (ESCEO) published an algorithm that further divide the high-risk category into high- and very-high-risk classifications [10]. To this end, a fracture probability that exceeds the intervention threshold by 20% would identify individuals with very high risk of fracture [7, 10]. The patient reported here had a history of previous fragility fracture, which according with the majority of guidelines worldwide can be considered for treatment without the need for further risk assessment. However, her 10-year probability of fracture was further assessed by FRAX. Interestingly, although the patient's BMD was not in the osteoporotic range, her 10-year probability of fracture exceeded the country-specific intervention threshold by 20%, identifying this patient as having a very-high risk of fracture [10]. This approach could not only define the need for pharmacological intervention but also guide the choice of the initial anti-osteoporotic agent and the duration of therapy [9, 10].

Additional fracture risk tools such as Garvan Fracture Risk Calculator and QFracture risk calculator are also available, but they were developed based on data from single countries, limiting their use worldwide [11, 12].

In addition to clinical risk factors, skeletal features other than areal BMD contribute to overall fracture risk. Bone geometry, microarchitecture, microdamage, rate of bone turnover, and mineralization contribute to bone strength and risk of fracture [13–15]. However, methodologies that evaluate bone strength independent of BMD are not readily available, being currently used as research tools. A major challenge, therefore, has been to develop a clinically available tool that permits evaluation of skeletal structure beyond BMD by DXA. To this end, TBS was developed as another approach for assessing skeletal bone structure noninvasively from DXA projection images [16]. TBS (unitless) is a gray-level texture measure that provides an indirect index of bone architecture [17, 18]. It is measured at the lumbar spine with specialized software (TBS iNsight®, MedImaps) that uses the same region of interest as conventional BMD measurement [19]. Of note, TBS can be artefactually reduced by excessive abdominal soft tissue [20, 21] and should not be measured in individuals with BMI outside of the range 15–37 kg/m^2 [17].

TBS predicts the risk of fracture independent of BMD by DXA and clinical risk factors [22–26]. The International Society for Clinical Densitometry (ISCD) and the ESCEO support the use of TBS to assess fracture risk in postmenopausal women and older men [27, 28]. However, although a low TBS is associated with greater risk of fracture, a TBS threshold to initiate treatment has not been defined, and TBS should not be used as a single measurement to guide treatment decisions [27]. Alternatively, TBS can be entered in the FRAX calculator online, allowing for the calculation of TBS-adjusted 10-year probability of fracture, assisting in treatment decisions (Fig. 3.1). In general, the use of TBS to adjust the FRAX score has a lower impact with increasing age, and a greater clinical effect in those patients who are close to the intervention threshold by FRAX without TBS [19].

There is no consensus regarding what represents low versus normal TBS values, but a metanalyses involving 17,809 men and women from 14 prospective population-based cohorts from North America, Asia, Australia, and Europe described TBS thresholds of 1.23 and 1.31 using a tertile analysis. Patients whose TBS was lower than 1.23 presented a high fracture risk, while those with TBS between 1.23 and 1.31 had an intermediate risk, and individuals with TBS greater than 1.31 had the lowest fracture risk. The patient reported here had a TBS of 1.11, which would indicate a high fracture risk. The use of TBS to adjust the FRAX score in this case increased the 10-year probability of MOF by 62% and doubled the risk of hip fracture calculated by FRAX) without TBS (Fig. 3.1).

Management

According to the recently published Endocrine Society (ES) guidelines for the management of osteoporosis in postmenopausal women, the patient presented here would be considered at high risk for fracture and could be treated with a bisphosphonate [29, 30]. Women with vertebral fractures associated with a BMD T-score in the osteoporotic range are at very high risk of fracture and may be treated with bone-forming agents as the initial therapy [29, 30]. Accordingly, the IOF/ESCEO and the American Association of Clinical Endocrinologists (AACE) guidelines also support the use of osteoanabolic agents as the first line of treatment in such patients [9, 10]. There are differences between the guidelines with regard to classification of patients at very high risk. The AACE guideline suggests that patients at very-high risk of fracture include those with recent fracture (within the past 12 months), those who have fractures while on approved osteoporosis therapy, history of multiple fractures, fractures while on drugs that increase fracture risk (e.g., long-term glucocorticoids), those with a very low T-score (e.g., <−3.0), high risk of falls or history of injurious falls, and those with a very-high fracture probability by FRAX [9]. Similarly, the IOF/ESCEO guidelines use the FRAX score to categorize the risk of fracture, such that patients with a 10-year fracture probability that exceeds the intervention threshold by 20% would be classified at very high risk [10]. This is the case for the patient presented here, so that one could argue that she should have been treated with an osteoanabolic agent. However, the evidence supporting the superiority of anabolic agents over antiresorptive agents in reducing fracture risk was demonstrated in patients with very high fracture risk due to the presence of previous vertebral fractures and/or prolonged glucocorticoid use [31–33]. These risk factors were absent in the patient presented here, and initial treatment with alendronate was supported by the ES guidelines [29, 30].

The patient's treatment was monitored using BMD by DXA and serum CTX, whereas TBS was not reassessed. The 2019 ISCD Position Development Conference concluded that the role of TBS in monitoring antiresorptive therapy is unclear [34]. Several studies have shown minimal changes in TBS in patients treated with bisphosphonates or denosumab for up to 3 years, with the majority of patients presenting a TBS improvement much lower than the least significant change [27, 34]. The use of TBS for monitoring patients on osteoanabolic therapy may be useful [27].

Some guidelines recommend FRAX reassessment in patients on bisphosphonates to define the duration of treatment and suggest a drug holiday in individuals whose FRAX risk falls below the intervention threshold [35]. This approach, however, has limitations, since the 10-year FRAX-probabilities of fracture can be overestimated in patients on osteoporosis treatment [36].

Outcome

The patient increased her calcium intake to 1200 mg/day, including 500 mg of calcium supplements, started on vitamin D_3 supplementation to maintain 25-hydroxyvitamin D levels >30 ng/mL and was treated with alendronate 70 mg weekly. At approximately 3 months on treatment, her serum 25-hydroxyvitamin D was 31.8 ng/mL, and her serum CTX was at 0.165 ng/mL, representing a decline of 63% compared to the baseline measurement, indicating a satisfactory level of compliance and good response to treatment. The BMD by DXA 1 year following treatment remained stable, with a nonsignificant change of +1.2% at the lumbar spine, and +2.2% at the total hip. The patient is now on year 4 of treatment, without incident fractures.

Clinical Pearls and Pitfalls
- Skeletal features other than BMD by DXA, as well as extraskeletal risk factors, contribute to overall fracture risk and should be identified to better select patients for anti-osteoporotic treatment.
- FRAX uses readily assessable clinical risk factors, with or without BMD, to estimate 10-year probabilities of major osteoporotic fractures and hip fractures, with the adoption of country-specific thresholds to guide treatment decisions.
- FRAX can be used without BMD, although the use of clinical risk factors in conjunction with BMD improves fracture prediction, particularly in the case of hip fractures.
- Limitations of FRAX include the lack of validation in patients on anti-osteoporotic treatment; the use of T-score at the femoral neck only, disregarding other sites (e.g., lumbar spine); lack of dose response for several risk factors (e.g., number of prior vertebral fractures); and the absence of important clinical risk factors such as history of falls.
- Trabecular bone score (TBS) is a gray-level textural measurement derived from lumbar spine DXA images that provides an indirect index of bone architecture and predicts the risk of fracture, independent of BMD by DXA and clinical risk factors.
- TBS can be entered into the FRAX calculator online, allowing for the calculation of TBS-adjusted 10-year probability of fracture, assisting in treatment decisions.
- The role of TBS in monitoring antiresorptive therapy is unclear.

References

1. Wainwright SA, Marshall LM, Ensrud KE, Cauley JA, Black DM, Hillier TA, et al. Hip fracture in women without osteoporosis. J Clin Endocrinol Metab. 2005;90(5):2787–93.
2. Siris ES, Miller PD, Barrett-Connor E, Faulkner KG, Wehren LE, Abbott TA, et al. Identification and fracture outcomes of undiagnosed low bone mineral density in postmenopausal women: results from the National Osteoporosis Risk Assessment. JAMA. 2001;286(22):2815–22.
3. Kanis JA, Oden A, Johnell O, Johansson H, De Laet C, Brown J, et al. The use of clinical risk factors enhances the performance of BMD in the prediction of hip and osteoporotic fractures in men and women. Osteoporos Int. 2007;18(8):1033–46.
4. Leslie WD, Lix LM, Johansson H, Oden A, McCloskey E, Kanis JA, et al. Independent clinical validation of a Canadian FRAX tool: fracture prediction and model calibration. J Bone Miner Res. 2010;25(11):2350–8.
5. Hillier TA, Cauley JA, Rizzo JH, Pedula KL, Ensrud KE, Bauer DC, et al. WHO absolute fracture risk models (FRAX): do clinical risk factors improve fracture prediction in older women without osteoporosis? J Bone Miner Res. 2011;26(8):1774–82.
6. Tamaki J, Iki M, Kadowaki E, Sato Y, Kajita E, Kagamimori S, et al. Fracture risk prediction using FRAX(R): a 10-year follow-up survey of the Japanese Population-Based Osteoporosis (JPOS) Cohort Study. Osteoporos Int. 2011;22(12):3037–45.
7. Kanis JA, Harvey NC, Johansson H, Liu E, Vandenput L, Lorentzon M, et al. A decade of FRAX: how has it changed the management of osteoporosis? Aging Clin Exp Res. 2020;32(2):187–96.
8. Liu J, Curtis EM, Cooper C, Harvey NC. State of the art in osteoporosis risk assessment and treatment. J Endocrinol Investig. 2019;42(10):1149–64.
9. Camacho PM, Petak SM, Binkley N, Diab DL, Eldeiry LS, Farooki A, et al. American Association of Clinical Endocrinologists/American College of Endocrinology Clinical Practice Guidelines for the diagnosis and treatment of postmenopausal osteoporosis-2020 update. Endocr Pract. 2020;26(Suppl 1):1–46.
10. Kanis JA, Harvey NC, McCloskey E, Bruyere O, Veronese N, Lorentzon M, et al. Algorithm for the management of patients at low, high and very high risk of osteoporotic fractures. Osteoporos Int. 2020;31(1):1–12.
11. Hippisley-Cox J, Coupland C. Derivation and validation of updated QFracture algorithm to predict risk of osteoporotic fracture in primary care in the United Kingdom: prospective open cohort study. BMJ. 2012;344:e3427.

12. Nguyen ND, Frost SA, Center JR, Eisman JA, Nguyen TV. Development of prognostic nomograms for individualizing 5-year and 10-year fracture risks. Osteoporos Int. 2008;19(10):1431–44.
13. Nishiyama KK, Macdonald HM, Hanley DA, Boyd SK. Women with previous fragility fractures can be classified based on bone microarchitecture and finite element analysis measured with HR-pQCT. Osteoporos Int. 2013;24(5):1733–40.
14. Garnero P, Hausherr E, Chapuy MC, Marcelli C, Grandjean H, Muller C, et al. Markers of bone resorption predict hip fracture in elderly women: the EPIDOS Prospective Study. J Bone Miner Res. 1996;11(10):1531–8.
15. Sroga GE, Vashishth D. Effects of bone matrix proteins on fracture and fragility in osteoporosis. Curr Osteoporos Rep. 2012;10(2):141–50.
16. Hans D, Barthe N, Boutroy S, Pothuaud L, Winzenrieth R, Krieg MA. Correlations between trabecular bone score, measured using antero-posterior dual-energy X-ray absorptiometry acquisition, and 3-dimensional parameters of bone microarchitecture: an experimental study on human cadaver vertebrae. J Clin Densitom. 2011;14(3):302–12.
17. Silva BC, Leslie WD. Trabecular bone score: a new DXA-derived measurement for fracture risk assessment. Endocrinol Metab Clin N Am. 2017;46(1):153–80.
18. Silva BC, Leslie WD, Resch H, Lamy O, Lesnyak O, Binkley N, et al. Trabecular bone score: a noninvasive analytical method based upon the DXA image. J Bone Miner Res. 2014;29(3):518–30.
19. Silva BC, Leslie WD. Trabecular bone score. In: Primer on the metabolic bone diseases and disorders of mineral metabolism. Hoboken: Wiley; 2018. p. 277–86.
20. Kim JH, Choi HJ, Ku EJ, Hong AR, Kim KM, Kim SW, et al. Regional body fat depots differently affect bone microarchitecture in postmenopausal Korean women. Osteoporos Int. 2016;27(3):1161–8.
21. Looker AC, Sarafrazi Isfahani N, Fan B, Shepherd JA. Trabecular bone scores and lumbar spine bone mineral density of US adults: comparison of relationships with demographic and body size variables. Osteoporos Int. 2016;27(8):2467–75.
22. Boutroy S, Hans D, Sornay-Rendu E, Vilayphiou N, Winzenrieth R, Chapurlat R. Trabecular bone score improves fracture risk prediction in non-osteoporotic women: the OFELY study. Osteoporos Int. 2013;24(1):77–85.
23. Briot K, Paternotte S, Kolta S, Eastell R, Reid DM, Felsenberg D, et al. Added value of trabecular bone score to bone mineral density for prediction of osteoporotic fractures in postmenopausal women: the OPUS study. Bone. 2013;57(1):232–6.
24. Hans D, Goertzen AL, Krieg MA, Leslie WD. Bone microarchitecture assessed by TBS predicts osteoporotic fractures independent of bone density: the Manitoba study. J Bone Miner Res. 2011;26(11):2762–9.

25. McCloskey EV, Oden A, Harvey NC, Leslie WD, Hans D, Johansson H, et al. A meta-analysis of trabecular bone score in fracture risk prediction and its relationship to FRAX. J Bone Miner Res. 2016;31(5):940–8.
26. Schousboe JT, Vo T, Taylor BC, Cawthon PM, Schwartz AV, Bauer DC, et al. Prediction of incident major osteoporotic and hip fractures by trabecular bone score (TBS) and prevalent radiographic vertebral fracture in older men. J Bone Miner Res. 2016;31(3):690–7.
27. Silva BC, Broy SB, Boutroy S, Schousboe JT, Shepherd JA, Leslie WD. Fracture risk prediction by non-BMD DXA measures: the 2015 ISCD official positions part 2: trabecular bone score. J Clin Densitom. 2015;18(3):309–30.
28. Harvey NC, Gluer CC, Binkley N, McCloskey EV, Brandi ML, Cooper C, et al. Trabecular bone score (TBS) as a new complementary approach for osteoporosis evaluation in clinical practice. Bone. 2015;78:216–24.
29. Eastell R, Rosen CJ, Black DM, Cheung AM, Murad MH, Shoback D. Pharmacological management of osteoporosis in postmenopausal women: an Endocrine Society* clinical practice guideline. J Clin Endocrinol Metab. 2019;104(5):1595–622.
30. Shoback D, Rosen CJ, Black DM, Cheung AM, Murad MH, Eastell R. Pharmacological management of osteoporosis in postmenopausal women: an Endocrine Society guideline update. J Clin Endocrinol Metab. 2020;105(3):dgaa048.
31. Saag KG, Petersen J, Brandi ML, Karaplis AC, Lorentzon M, Thomas T, et al. Romosozumab or alendronate for fracture prevention in women with osteoporosis. N Engl J Med. 2017;377(15):1417–27.
32. Kendler DL, Marin F, Zerbini CAF, Russo LA, Greenspan SL, Zikan V, et al. Effects of teriparatide and risedronate on new fractures in postmenopausal women with severe osteoporosis (VERO): a multicentre, double-blind, double-dummy, randomised controlled trial. Lancet. 2018;391(10117):230–40.
33. Saag KG, Shane E, Boonen S, Marin F, Donley DW, Taylor KA, et al. Teriparatide or alendronate in glucocorticoid-induced osteoporosis. N Engl J Med. 2007;357(20):2028–39.
34. Krohn K, Schwartz EN, Chung YS, Lewiecki EM. Dual-energy X-ray absorptiometry monitoring with trabecular bone score: 2019 ISCD official position. J Clin Densitom. 2019;22(4):501–5.
35. Adler RA, El-Hajj Fuleihan G, Bauer DC, Camacho PM, Clarke BL, Clines GA, et al. Managing osteoporosis in patients on long-term bisphosphonate treatment: report of a Task Force of the American Society for Bone and Mineral Research. J Bone Miner Res. 2016;31(1):16–35.
36. Leslie WD, Lix LM, Johansson H, Oden A, McCloskey E, Kanis JA, et al. Does osteoporosis therapy invalidate FRAX for fracture prediction? J Bone Miner Res. 2012;27(6):1243–51.

Steroids, Aromatase Inhibitors, and Other Drugs Associated with Osteoporosis

4

Guido Zavatta and Bart L. Clarke

Case Presentation

A 55-year-old woman is referred for newly diagnosed postmenopausal osteoporosis, without previous fractures. She was simulta-
neously diagnosed with giant cell arteritis and advised to take
prednisone 60 mg a day for 1 month by her rheumatologist, with
a slow taper planned over the next 6 months. Her bone mineral
density test showed her lowest T-score to be −2.9 at her lumbar
spine, with her hip T-scores ranging from −2.1 at her left femur
neck to −2.5 at her right total hip site.

She has not previously taken antiresorptive or osteoanabolic
therapy. She underwent spontaneous menopause at age 48 years
and did not take hormone therapy due to lack of hot flashes. Her
comorbidities include significant gastroesophageal reflux disease
(GERD) not responding to omeprazole, celiac disease on a gluten-
free diet, and hypertension on metoprolol and lisinopril.

Her total daily calcium intake is 1200 mg elemental calcium
through her dietary intake of 600 mg elemental calcium and sup-

G. Zavatta · B. L. Clarke (✉)
Mayo Clinic E18-A, Rochester, MN, USA
e-mail: guido.zavatta2@unibo.it; clarke.bart@mayo.edu

© The Author(s), under exclusive license to Springer Nature
Switzerland AG 2021
N. E. Cusano (ed.), *Osteoporosis*,
https://doi.org/10.1007/978-3-030-83951-2_4

43

plemental calcium citrate 600 mg once a day. She takes vitamin D3 1000 IU once a day. Her laboratory studies show normal serum calcium, phosphorus, creatinine, eGFR, parathyroid hormone, and 25-hydroxyvitamin D levels. She exercises by walking 2 miles every day.

Given her high risk of future fracture, with anticipated high-dose glucocorticoid therapy for at least 6 months, and other medical comorbidities of GERD and celiac disease, consideration is given to antiresorptive therapy.

Management

Bone strength may be profoundly affected by a variety of medications that produce a negative balance in bone remodeling, leading to disproportionate resorption compared to bone formation, and enhanced fracture risk. Drug-induced fragility fractures may occur at different times or sites compared to those more typically seen in postmenopausal osteoporosis. Drug-induced osteoporosis may be more challenging to prevent or manage effectively because the offending agent(s) often cannot be replaced with equivalent drugs that have neutral effects on bone. This chapter focuses on glucocorticoids, aromatase inhibitors, and other common medications known to contribute to bone loss or fractures. This information may help improve clinical care of many patients, especially in primary care settings.

Glucocorticoids

Glucocorticoid-induced osteoporosis (GIOP) is the most frequent cause of secondary osteoporosis. Glucocorticoids are normally used to treat a wide variety of chronic medical conditions. In the United States, it is estimated that 1.0% of the population (2.5 million people) aged 20 years or older routinely receive glucocorticoids [1]. Fragility fractures due to glucocorticoid exposure may also occur in the setting of endogenous glucocorticoid overproduction by the adrenal glands in Cushing's syndrome, both in overt and subclinical phenotypes [2].

Bone quality, in addition to bone mineral density, is affected in glucocorticoid-treated patients. Decreased bone formation with an imbalance toward bone resorption are thought to be the main mechanisms sustaining bone loss over time, with osteoblast and osteocyte apoptosis observed at the cellular level. Osteoclast recruitment increases during the first 6–12 months of exposure, leading to a transient increase in bone resorption soon after therapy is started. At the molecular level, increased release of receptor activator of nuclear factor kappa-B ligand (RANKL) by osteoblasts increases the RANKL/osteoprotegerin ratio above 1.0, leading to progressive stimulation in osteoclast activity and increased bone turnover. Glucocorticoid therapy causes persistently decreased bone formation during prolonged use. The combination of these effects leads to significant and rapid bone loss.

These changes may be monitored using bone turnover markers. Knowledge of these markers may help guide treatment of patients with either antiresorptive or osteoanabolic agents. N-terminal propeptide of type 1 collagen and bone-specific alkaline phosphatase are serum markers of osteoblast activity that are usually decreased during long-term glucocorticoid treatment, and that increase after withdrawal of glucocorticoid therapy. These markers also increase markedly in response to osteoanabolic therapy. By contrast, serum C-telopeptide is expected to moderately increase during the first several months of glucocorticoid administration, and then return to normal with long-term therapy. Osteocalcin, a mixed marker of both bone formation and resorption, is typically low or suppressed during long-term glucocorticoid therapy. Sclerostin, produced by osteocytes and osteoblasts, is an inhibitor of the Wnt-signaling pathway that is usually decreased due to a reduction in osteocyte number caused by glucocorticoid therapy [3].

The detrimental effects of glucocorticoids on bone are rapid, thereby making bone density less useful in promptly identifying patients at high risk for fractures. However, BMD by DXA is still acknowledged to be the best tool for monitoring effectiveness of osteoporosis treatment. In GIOP, trabecular bone is affected more by glucocorticoid therapy than cortical bone. Recent advances in technology may aid in detecting early damage to the bone microarchitecture. Trabecular bone score (TBS) has been shown to predict fracture risk independently of DXA during glucocorticoid therapy. This proprietary software device (TBS Insight®, Medimaps, Meriganc, France) is used to assess skeletal microarchitecture by evaluating the gray-scale texture of lumbar spine DXA images. TBS has been included in the FRAX algorithm to further guide treatment decisions [4].

Dose, duration, and route of administration of glucocorticoids should all be considered when evaluating increased fracture risk in this setting. Vertebral fractures are the most common fractures reported in patients with GIOP. Fracture risk is significantly increased as early as 3 months after the start of glucocorticoid therapy and peaks at around 12 months of therapy [1]. Fracture incidence decreases rapidly after cessation of glucocorticoids regardless of the preceding cumulative dose. Reduction in fracture risk can be detected as early as 3–12 months after the discontinuation of glucocorticoids. Daily dose of glucocorticoids is correlated to fracture risk. Patients receiving greater than 7.5 mg of prednisolone equivalent each day have more than a twofold increased risk of vertebral or hip fracture compared to those taking less than 2.5 mg each day. Patients receiving 2.5–7.5 mg of prednisolone equivalent each day may have at least a 50% increase in risk of vertebral and hip fractures compared to those taking less than 2.5 mg/day. Prednisolone equivalent doses as low as 2.5 mg per day have been associated with a relative risk of fracture of 1.17 (95% CI; 1.10–1.25) for nonvertebral fractures, and 1.55 (95% CI; 1.20–2.01) for vertebral fractures, although some of this increased risk may be due to systemic inflammation not fully suppressed by low-dose glucocorticoid therapy [5].

Intermittent use of high-dose oral glucocorticoids (>15 mg/day) has been associated with increased risk of fragility fractures, but not specifically hip fractures, as long as the cumulative exposure remains less than 1.0 g. When cumulative exposure is >5 g, a substantial increase in fracture risk is seen in spite of intermittent exposure, more like what is seen with continuous daily treatment [6]. FRAX estimates are most accurate when doses of glucocorticoids range between 2.5 and 7.5 mg/day. To further improve accuracy, FRAX risk may be adjusted downward by 20%, or upward by 15%, if doses are below or above these thresholds [7].

Optimization of calcium intake through diet and/or supplements and maintenance of serum 25-hydroxyvitamin D > 30 ng/mL are recommended during glucocorticoid therapy. The 2011 National Academy of Medicine (previously the Institute of Medicine) report advised that the recommended daily allowance (RDA) of calcium be 1200 mg through diet and supplements and that the vitamin D RDA be 600–800 IU.

The Food and Drug Administration has approved five medications for treatment of GIOP based on improvements in BMD alone from placebo-controlled trials, without fracture data (Table 4.1). These drugs include oral alendronate 5 mg/day for men and premenopausal women, and 10 mg/day for postmeno-

Table 4.1 Therapeutic options for treatment of glucocorticoid- or aromatase inhibitor-induced bone loss

Treatment	Glucocorticoid-induced osteoporosis	Aromatase inhibitor-induced bone loss
Alendronate 10 mg po each day	Improves BMD and reduces vertebral fracture risk	Improves BMD
Risedronate 5 mg po each day	Improves BMD and reduces vertebral fracture risk	Improves BMD
Ibandronate 150 mg po each month	No data	Improves BMD
Zoledronate 5 mg IV each year	Improves BMD	Improves BMD when given as 4 mg IV twice each year
Denosumab 60 mg SC every 6 months	Improves BMD	Improves BMD and reduces fractures (fractures independent of BMD)
Teriparatide 20 mcg SC each day	Improves BMD and reduces fracture risk	Not recommended
Abaloparatide 80 mcg SC each day	No data available. Currently approved only for postmenopausal osteoporosis.	Not recommended
Romosozumab 210 mg SC each month for 12 months	No data available	No data available

pausal women not receiving estrogen therapy; oral risedronate 5 mg/day; intravenous zoledronic acid 5 mg once annually; subcutaneously injected denosumab 60 mg every 6 months; and subcutaneously injected teriparatide 20 mcg/day. No data are available as yet for abaloparatide or romosozumab in GIOP. At present, the high cost of these medications favors the bisphosphonates as first-line agents, although the pathophysiological mechanisms causing GIOP justify more widespread use of PTH analogs as initial therapy [8].

Aromatase Inhibitors and Other Endocrine Therapies in Breast Cancer

Up to one in eight women will develop breast cancer during their lifetime. Most breast cancers express estrogen receptors, and women with these cancers are therefore candidates for hormone therapy with medications that suppress the production or action of estrogens on estrogen receptors. Aromatase inhibitors (AIs), along with gonadotropin-releasing hormone (GnRH) analogs and tamoxifen, are the mainstays of hormonal treatment. All these drugs except tamoxifen in postmenopausal women have adverse effects on the skeleton, because they interfere with estrogen production or estrogen signaling [9].

AIs inhibit the aromatase enzyme (CYP19A1), which converts androgens to estrogens within breast cancer cells. AIs also decrease estrogen production from adipose tissue, thereby reducing estrogen levels in the circulation by 80–95% in postmenopausal women [10]. There are two types of AIs: steroidal (exemestane) and nonsteroidal (anastrozole and letrozole), depending on the chemical structure of the molecule. Exemestane yields an active metabolite, 17-hydroxyexemestane, which binds tightly to the androgen receptor, possibly causing signaling through the androgen receptor. To date there is no evidence whether this may attenuate the negative effects of this drug on bone metabolism. GnRH analogs act on the pituitary to inhibit the pituitary-gonadal axis, thereby decreasing release of luteinizing hormone and suppressing estrogen production by the ovaries.

Tamoxifen is a selective-estrogen receptor modulator (SERM), with antagonist properties on breast and cancer tissue. Management of estrogen receptor-positive breast cancer differs according to menopausal status.

In premenopausal women, the ovaries are the main source of estrogens, and the goal of cancer therapy is to suppress ovarian estrogen production with GnRH analogs, with subsequent treatment with AIs to prevent non-ovarian estrogen production. In premenopausal women, the use of tamoxifen has been associated with excessive bone loss due to interference with estrogen [11]. However, tamoxifen co-administered with GnRH analogs may partially attenuate GnRH analog-induced bone loss due to beneficial effects of tamoxifen on bone in the absence of high circulating levels of endogenous estrogen [12].

There are limited data on spontaneous bone loss in young women undergoing menopause for reasons other than cancer chemotherapy or oophorectomy. It appears that younger women undergoing menopause lose bone very rapidly, at a rate of up to 10% per year, regardless of the underlying cause of estrogen deprivation [13]. Despite this, fracture data are lacking, possibly because this group is at lower baseline risk for fracture due to their younger age and possibly higher body mass index.

When AIs are used to treat premenopausal women, BMD loss is rapid at both the spine, with up to 11.3% loss over 36 months, and the hip, with up to 7.3% loss at 36 months [12].This observation has led to the recommendation to evaluate for bone loss even at younger ages and to monitor changes in BMD with sequential DXA.

In postmenopausal women, the goal of adjuvant cancer therapy is mainly to suppress non-ovarian estrogen production. This is successfully achieved with AIs, which are currently first-line therapy. If these drugs are not tolerated, then tamoxifen is used to reduce the risk of breast cancer recurrence. Tamoxifen increases BMD, while AIs result in stimulation of bone resorption and consequently bone loss. The effect of AIs on BMD in postmenopausal women is well characterized, although the lack of a control group without AI treatment limits the interpretation of fracture data compared to postmenopausal women of the same age. This may partially explain some of the differences in management strategies between European and American guidelines [14, 15].

Table 4.2 summarizes the major clinical trials conducted with AIs in postmenopausal women. It is important to note that AIs have mostly been compared to tamoxifen, which may magnify the perceived negative effect of AIs on bone loss or fractures because tamoxifen typically increases bone density. None of the clinical trials used fractures as a main endpoint, with fractures reported as adverse events. There was substantial heterogeneity of fractures across study groups, typically running at 5–10% at 5 years of treatment. In the first year of AI therapy, bone loss is higher than the expected physiological BMD loss for postmenopausal women, while further bone loss seems to slow somewhat thereafter. With longer treatment with AIs, fractures are expected to increase further. This supports the use of antiresorptive agents early after initiation of AI therapy to prevent AI-induced bone loss. Data from the clinical trials may underestimate the real fracture incidence, because osteoporosis was often an exclusion criterion for study participation. However, a recent population-based study using the Manitoba registry in Manitoba, Canada, found that AI-treated women did not have substantially increased fractured risk [16]. More data on fractures in real-world settings are needed. Women starting AI therapy should be evaluated for bone loss and risk factors for fracture, treated accordingly, and monitored for bone loss periodically until they stop therapy.

While there is agreement that bone health should be evaluated in women starting treatment with AIs, consensus has not yet been achieved regarding the threshold for starting antiresorptive treatment.

The 2020 guidelines by the European Society for Medical Oncology [14] support intervention in most AI-treated patients. Clinical risk factors and BMD are recommended to guide clinicians on whether to start antiresorptive therapy (see Table 4.1 for available medications). BMD T-scores below −2.0 are an indication for antiresorptive treatment. BMD T-scores below −1.5 should be used to start treatment if accompanied by other clinical risk factors for fracture.

Table 4.2 Major clinical trials with aromatase inhibitors

Aromatase inhibitor	Comparator	Age at study entry (years)	Change in lumbar spine BMD (%)	New onset of osteoporosis (%)	Clinical fractures (%)
Letrozole					
MA.17R (AIs for 10 years) Median follow-up of 6.3 years	Placebo	65.6	In sub-protocol MA.17: N = 226, follow-up 1.6 years: −5.35% vs. −0.71%	11% vs. 6% (vs. placebo) (P < 0.001) (by DXA)	14% vs. 9%
NSABP B-42	Placebo	<60, 34%[a]	NR	4.0 vs. 3.4 (vs. placebo) (P = 0.29)	5.4 vs. 4.8% (P = NS) (over 7 years)
IDEAL (2.5 years)	Placebo	<55, 27.5%	NR	7.5%	2.8%
IDEAL (5 years)	Placebo	<55, 28.5%	NR	12.7%	5.0%
BIG 1–98	Tamoxifen (sequential treatment, see Fig. 4.1)	61.9	NR	Prevalence of LS and TH osteoporosis highest on tamoxifen (for 2 years), followed by letrozole (for 3 years) (14.5% vs. 7.1%) at 60 months	9.3% vs. 6.5% (over 60 months)

(continued)

Table 4.2 (continued)

Aromatase inhibitor	Comparator	Age at study entry (years)	Change in lumbar spine BMD (%)	New onset of osteoporosis (%)	Clinical fractures (%)
Anastrozole					
DATA, years 0–3	Anastrozole for 3 years, after tamoxifen	57.6 <60, 58%	N = 308 (subgroup at 2 years): −4.1% vs. +2.2%	16.4%	7.6%
DATA, years 0–6	Anastrozole for 6 years, after tamoxifen	57.6 <60, 58%	−0.075 was mean reduction in LS T-score/year on Anastrozole (1%/year)	20.9%	10.0%
ABCSG 16 (2 years)	–	<80	–	–	4.7%
ABCSG 16 (5 years)	–	<80	–	–	6.3%
ATAC (subgroup N = 197)	Tamoxifen	64	−6.1% vs. +2.8% after 5 years (−2.3% vs. +1.4% at 1 year)	No patients with normal BMD at baseline became osteoporotic at 5 years	NR
ATAC (N = 6186)	Tamoxifen	64	–	–	11% vs. 7.7% all fractures (vertebral 1.5% vs. 0.9%, sites other than femur or wrist 7.1% vs. 4.6%)

Exemestane					
IES (exemestane after 2–3 years of tamoxifen)	Tamoxifen	64.2	−4.0% (−2.7% within 6 months) vs. −0.6% at 24 months (subgroup with data on bone outcomes)	No patient with normal BMD at baseline developed osteoporosis (subgroup with data on bone outcomes)	7.0% vs. 5.0% at 58 months
TEAM-GER	Tamoxifen	61	−2.8% (−2.6% within 6 months) vs. +0.5% at 1 year ($P = 0.0008$)	2/78 vs. 3/83 with osteoporosis at 12 months	–
Physiologic bone loss at lumbar spine					
Early menopause			Up to 2%/year		
Late menopause			Up to 1%/year		
Normal aging			0.5–1%/year		

These clinical trials were not designed to study the impact of these drugs on bone metabolism. Osteoporosis was often an exclusionary criterion, so study populations were all at low risk for fractures at baseline. Fractures were reported by patients as adverse events and treatment of osteoporosis was not standardized, so that some patients could have been on bisphosphonates during the trials. Tamoxifen in the comparator group might have falsely elevated the perceived adjunctive fracture risk of aromatase inhibitors in these studies because it protects against bone loss in postmenopausal women

Abbreviations: BMD bone mineral density, DXA dual-energy X-ray absorptiometry, LS lumbar spine, NR not recorded, TH total hip

[a]Proportion of patients with age less than indicated

In comparison, the 2019 guidelines by the American Society of Clinical Oncology [15] recommend starting antiresorptive treatment if patients have osteoporosis or prior history of fractures, or if the FRAX estimates are $\geq 3\%$ for hip fracture or $\geq 20\%$ for major osteoporotic fracture in patients with osteopenia.

Both guidelines agree that women starting AI therapy should receive proper counseling regarding bone health and calcium and vitamin D intake. They both recommend that BMD should be monitored every 2 years, or more often if the results would influence clinical decisions.

Bone density tends to improve after AI treatment is completed. BMD tends to recover [12], although it may not return to baseline after prolonged treatment for more than 5 years (Fig. 4.1).

Clinical Practice Points and Open Questions Regarding AIs

- There is no specific recommendation on the duration of antiresorptive therapy or whether bisphosphonate holidays should be considered, especially when patients may continue treatment with AIs for up to 10 years.
- Denosumab should always be followed by bisphosphonates to prevent rebound bone loss and/or vertebral fractures.
- The reasons for treatment with antiresorptive agents to prevent AI-induced bone loss should be explained to patients at the commencement of AI therapy.
- Bisphosphonates or denosumab may be used by oncologists adjunctively to help prevent skeletal metastasis of breast cancer in postmenopausal women [17].

Other Medications Associated with Osteoporosis

Many other drugs have been associated with bone loss or fractures, although most data are derived from observational studies, and causal association is more difficult to prove. However, all medications used by patients should be reviewed at diagnosis and

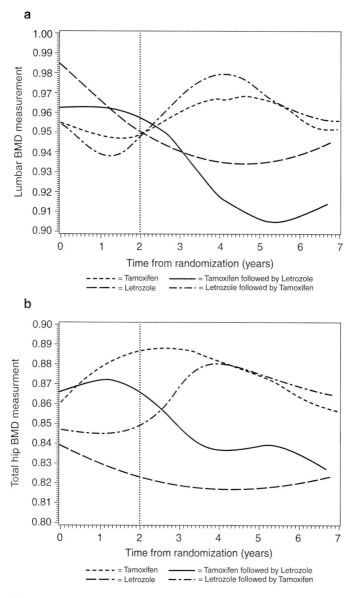

Fig. 4.1 Evolution of bone mineral density ((**a**) Lumbar spine, (**b**) Total hip) over time in patients sequentially treated with tamoxifen or letrozole in the BIG 1–98 trial. Age at study entry was 61 years. (Used with permission from Zaman et al. [24])

during monitoring for treatment of osteoporosis. The negative impact of several common medications on bone metabolism is reviewed here, with a more comprehensive list of drugs associated with bone loss presented in Table 4.3.

Men treated with *androgen deprivation therapy* (ADT) are at risk for bone loss and fracture. GnRH analogs such as leuprolide and anti-androgenic therapies such as cyproterone acetate, flutamide, and bicalutamide promote bone loss. Decreased endogenous testosterone production causes a reduction in circulating estradiol levels as well. Deceased serum 17β-estradiol is strongly associated with BMD loss in men, as it is in women. Patients treated with ADT should have bone density testing at the start of therapy, with a full clinical evaluation for fracture risk. Men with prior fragility fractures, T-scores ≤ −2.5, or FRAX-estimated 10-year hip fracture risk ≥3.0% or major osteoporotic fracture risk ≥20% should be treated with an antiresorptive medication. Bisphosphonates and denosumab have both been shown to prevent bone loss in randomized clinical trials, with denosumab effective at lowering vertebral fracture incidence [18].

Proton pump inhibitors (PPIs) have been shown to increase risk of hip fractures. Increased fall risk, impaired calcium absorption from the intestines due to reduced stomach acid production, and reduced solubilization of calcium carbonate (but not calcium citrate) have been suggested as potential mechanisms [19]. The overall data are not sufficiently strong to recommend avoidance of PPI used in patients with osteoporosis being treated with an antiresorptive or osteoanabolic medication.

Selective serotonin receptor uptake inhibitors (SSRIs) have been reported to increase fracture risk and bone loss in both women and men. The underlying mechanism is not yet clear but may be related to inhibition of Wnt signaling [20] after interaction with LRP-5.

Certain antidiabetic medications have been associated with fractures. *Thiazolidinediones* (TZDs) activate adipose tissue PPAR-γ, thereby reducing insulin resistance. The exact mechanism by which TZDs negatively affect the skeleton is unknown, but it is presumed related to inhibition of osteoblastic differentiation, thereby impairing bone formation. It is advisable to avoid

Table 4.3 Medications associated with osteoporosis or osteomalacia

Type of bone damage	Medication	Mechanism
Bone loss	Glucocorticoids	Decreased bone formation; early transient increase in bone resorption, sustained chronic normal bone resorption
	Aromatase inhibitors	Inhibit aromatase (CYP19A1), which converts androgens to estrogens, thereby reducing circulating estrogen
	Gonadotropin-releasing hormone (GnRH) analogues	Reduce GnRH release from the hypothalamus, suppressing LH- and FSH-induced activity in the ovaries (estrogen production) or testicles (androgen production). Estrogen levels from the ovaries or aromatase conversion are markedly reduced in both sexes
	Medroxyprogesterone acetate	Negative feedback on the pituitary results in decreased estrogen production
	Androgen deprivation therapy for prostate cancer	Suppresses androgen and estrogen levels. Effects on bone are due to estrogen depletion
	Tamoxifen in premenopausal women	Competes with endogenous estrogens for the estrogen receptor
	Thyroxine over-replacement	Increased bone turnover
	Thiazolidinediones	Activation of PPARγ increases marrow adiposity, increases insulin sensitivity, and reduces bone formation
	Canagliflozin	Uncertain, but higher rates of peripheral fractures (possibly increased falls)
	Imatinib	Unclear, prolonged use associated with hyperparathyroidism and hypophosphatemia

(continued)

Table 4.3 (continued)

Type of bone damage	Medication	Mechanism
	Calcineurin inhibitors	Increase bone turnover, hypomagnesemia, hypercalciuria
	Proton pump inhibitors/ H_2 receptor blockers	Decrease dietary calcium absorption (and absorption of calcium carbonate supplements)
	Loop diuretics	Inhibit calcium reabsorption by the kidney
	Selective serotonin receptor uptake inhibitors (SSRI)	Possible interference with Wnt signaling pathway
	Heparin	Unknown
	Warfarin	Thought to impair osteocalcin γ-carboxylation by inhibiting vitamin K-dependent γ-glutamyl carboxylase localized in osteoblasts. Gamma-carboxylation is essential for affinity of osteocalcin to bone matrix. Non-vitamin K antagonist oral anticoagulants are associated with lower risk of osteoporosis compared to warfarin
	HIV (human immunodeficiency virus) therapy	Promotes osteoclastogenesis
Osteomalacia	Antiepileptic drugs (phenobarbital, phenytoin, carbamazepine, and valproic acid)	Accelerate vitamin D metabolism in the liver by induction of CYP3A4 enzyme
	Tenofovir (antiretroviral)	Phosphate wasting from the kidney due to acquired Fanconi's syndrome: hypophosphatemia and mild 1,25-dihydroxyvitamin D deficiency result
	Iron carboxymaltose infusions	Increase FGF-23, promoting phosphate wasting by the kidneys

TZDs in patients at elevated risk of falls or fractures. *Canagliflozin*, a sodium-glucose cotransporter-2 (SGLT-2) inhibitor, promotes glucose and sodium excretion through the kidneys. BMD loss and peripheral fractures were reported as adverse events in an early phase 3 clinical trial [21]. By contrast, a recent large population-based study did not find increased fracture risk in middle-aged patients compared to patients treated with GLP-1 receptor agonists [22]. More data are needed with other SGLT-2 inhibitors, but a reasonable approach in the meantime is to avoid the use of these medications in patients at very high risk of fracture.

Various *antiepileptic drugs* induce hepatic catabolism of vitamin D, potentially causing severe vitamin D depletion, which may lead to osteomalacia. In patients taking anti-seizure medications including phenobarbital, phenytoin, carbamazepine, and valproic acid, it is important to measure serum 25-hydroxyvitamin D levels periodically and to provide vitamin D supplementation adequate to keep these levels within the optimal range.

Tenofovir and *ferric carboxymaltose* may cause renal tubular phosphate loss, leading to hypophosphatemia and thereby cause undermineralization of bone leading to osteomalacia. *Tenofovir* is used to treat patients with chronic hepatitis B or HIV and has been associated with non-FGF-23-mediated hypophosphatemia. Infusions of *ferric carboxymaltose* are used to treat acute and chronic iron deficiency anemia. This form of parenteral iron is associated with frequent FGF-23-mediated hypophosphatemia and osteomalacia. FGF-23-mediated effects last for several weeks after a single infusion [23]. Phosphate levels should be monitored in these patients, and hypophosphatemia should not be mistakenly attributed to tumor-induced osteomalacia. Patients with unexplained hypophosphatemia should have a careful review of their recent medication use.

Outcome

The US FDA has approved alendronate, risedronate, zoledronic acid, denosumab, and teriparatide for treatment of glucocorticoid-induced osteoporosis. The patient was felt to not be a candidate for oral bisphosphonates due to her celiac disease and GERD not responding to omeprazole. Intravenous zoledronic acid 5 mg over 15 minutes once a year for 3 years was felt to be a reasonable option if tolerated.

The 2017 American College of Rheumatology Guidelines for the Prevention and Treatment of Glucocorticoid-Induced Osteoporosis [8] would assess this patient to be at high risk of fracture because of her postmenopausal status and her lowest bone density T-score of −2.9, even though she has not had a previous fracture. Given her limitations on the use of oral bisphosphonates, zoledronic acid is the first agent to consider. If she could not tolerate zoledronic acid, then denosumab or teriparatide would be considered.

She received her first dose of intravenous zoledronic acid on the same day she started prednisone 60 mg once a day and received two subsequent yearly doses. She tolerated zoledronic acid without side effect, and her renal function remained normal. Her prednisone was tapered successfully off over 2 years without recurrence of her giant cell arteritis. Her bone density T-scores increased to −2.3 at her lumbar spine, −1.8 at her left femur neck, and −2.0 at her right total hip over the 3 years of therapy. She had no low-trauma fractures during this interval. After 3 years, she discontinued intravenous zoledronic acid and continued her calcium and vitamin D intake. Her bone density test was to be rechecked in 2 years.

Clinical Pearls/Pitfalls
- Patients with osteoporosis or osteopenia should have a review of their medications at each encounter, focusing on medications that affect bone health, as this might spare them from future fractures.
- Glucocorticoids, aromatase inhibitors, and other medications may inadvertently cause bone loss.
- Implementation of a strategy to monitor bone density and start therapy when needed may help prevent fractures when the offending medications cannot be stopped or replaced.

References

1. Buckley L, Humphrey MB. Glucocorticoid-induced osteoporosis. N Engl J Med. 2018;379(26):2547–56.
2. Di Dalmazi G, Vicennati V, Rinaldi E, et al. Progressively increased patterns of subclinical cortisol hypersecretion in adrenal incidentalomas differently predict major metabolic and cardiovascular outcomes: a large cross-sectional study. Eur J Endocrinol. 2012;166(4):669–77.
3. Chotiyarnwong P, McCloskey E. Pathogenesis of glucocorticoid-induced osteoporosis and options for treatment. Nat Rev Endocrinol. 2020;16(8):437–47.
4. Martineau P, Leslie WD, Johansson H, et al. In which patients does lumbar spine trabecular bone score (TBS) have the largest effect? Bone. 2018;113:161–8.
5. van Staa TP, Leufkens HGM, Abenhaim L, Zhang B, Cooper C. Oral corticosteroids and fracture risk: relationship to daily and cumulative doses. Rheumatology. 2000;39(12):1383–9.
6. de Vries F, Bracke M, Leufkens HGM, Lammers JWJ, Cooper C, van Staa TP. Fracture risk with intermittent high-dose oral glucocorticoid therapy. Arthritis Rheum. 2007;56(1):208–14.
7. Kanis JA, Johansson H, Oden A, McCloskey E. Guidance for the adjustment of FRAX according to the dose of glucocorticoids. Osteoporos Int. 2011;22(3):809–16.
8. Buckley L, Guyatt G, Fink HA, et al. 2017 American College of Rheumatology guideline for the prevention and treatment of glucocorticoid-induced osteoporosis. Arthritis Rheumatol. 2017;69(8):1521–37.
9. Rachner TD, Coleman R, Hadji P, Hofbauer LC. Bone health during endocrine therapy for cancer. Lancet Diabetes Endocrinol. 2018;6(11):901–10.
10. Chien AJ, Goss PE. Aromatase inhibitors and bone health in women with breast cancer. J Clin Oncol. 2006;24(33):5305–12.
11. Bedatsova L, Drake MT. The skeletal impact of cancer therapies. Br J Clin Pharmacol. 2019;85(6):1161–8.
12. Gnant M, Mlineritsch B, Luschin-Ebengreuth G, et al. Adjuvant endocrine therapy plus zoledronic acid in premenopausal women with early-stage breast cancer: 5-year follow-up of the ABCSG-12 bone-mineral density substudy. Lancet Oncol. 2008;9(9):840–9.
13. Genant HK, Cann CE, Ettinger B, Gordan GS. Quantitative computed tomography of vertebral spongiosa: a sensitive method for detecting early bone loss after oophorectomy. Ann Intern Med. 1982;97(5):699–705.
14. Coleman R, Hadji P, Body JJ, et al. Bone health in cancer: ESMO clinical practice guidelines. Ann Oncol. 2020;31(12):1650–63.
15. Burstein HJ, Lacchetti C, Griggs JJ. Adjuvant endocrine therapy for women with hormone receptor–positive breast cancer: ASCO clinical practice guideline focused update. J Oncol Pract. 2019;15(2):106–7.

16. Leslie WD, Morin SN, Lix LM, et al. Performance of FRAX in women with breast cancer initiating aromatase inhibitor therapy: a registry-based cohort study. J Bone Miner Res. 2019;34(8):1428–35.

17. Coleman R. Bisphosphonates and breast cancer – from cautious palliation to saving lives. Bone. 2020;140:115570.

18. Smith MR, Egerdie B, Toriz NH, et al. Denosumab in men receiving androgen-deprivation therapy for prostate cancer. N Engl J Med. 2009;361(8):745–55.

19. Nguyen KD, Bagheri B, Bagheri H. Drug-induced bone loss: a major safety concern in Europe. Expert Opin Drug Saf. 2018;17(10):1005–14.

20. Warden SJ, Robling AG, Haney EM, Turner CH, Bliziotes MM. The emerging role of serotonin (5-hydroxytryptamine) in the skeleton and its mediation of the skeletal effects of low-density lipoprotein receptor-related protein 5 (LRP5). Bone. 2010;46(1):4–12.

21. Neal B, Perkovic V, Mahaffey KW, et al. Canagliflozin and cardiovascular and renal events in type 2 diabetes. N Engl J Med. 2017;377(7):644–57.

22. Fralick M, Kim SC, Schneeweiss S, Kim D, Redelmeier DA, Patorno E. Fracture risk after initiation of use of canagliflozin: a cohort study. Ann Intern Med. 2019;170(3):155–63.

23. Wolf M, Rubin J, Achebe M, et al. Effects of iron isomaltoside vs. ferric carboxymaltose on hypophosphatemia in iron-deficiency anemia: two randomized clinical trials. JAMA – J Am Med Assoc. 2020;323(5):432–43.

24. Zaman K, Thürlimann B, Huober J, et al. Bone mineral density in breast cancer patients treated with adjuvant letrozole, tamoxifen, or sequences of letrozole and tamoxifen in the BIG 1–98 study. Ann Oncol. 2012;23(6):1474–81.

Secondary Causes and Contributors to Osteoporosis

5

Laura E. Ryan and Steven W. Ing

Case Presentation

A 55-year-old woman was referred for evaluation and management of osteoporosis by her primary care provider after bone density screening (her first) showed DXA scan BMD T-scores of −3.0 and −1.9 at the lumbar spine and left femoral neck, respectively. The spine Z-score was −2.0. There was no personal or parental history of fragility fracture. There was no significant loss of height versus historical young adult height. She achieved menarche at age 11, had regular monthly menses lasting 3–4 days, had five pregnancies (two miscarriages, three deliveries), and underwent natural menopause at age 50, without menopausal hormone therapy. Dietary calcium in childhood was adequate. She was active at work as a physical therapist and enjoyed walking 4 days/week. She had tonsillectomy, Cesarean section × 3, and laparoscopy showing left ovarian cyst. She did not smoke cigarettes nor drink alcohol regularly. She took a calcium-vitamin D (600 mg–400 IU) supplement daily, multivitamin daily, and topical vaginal cream twice weekly. Examination revealed a well-appearing Caucasian woman,

L. E. Ryan (✉) · S. W. Ing
Division of Endocrinology, Diabetes and Metabolism, The Ohio State University Wexner Medical Center, Columbus, OH, USA
e-mail: laura.ryan@osumc.edu; steven.ing@osumc.edu

© The Author(s), under exclusive license to Springer Nature Switzerland AG 2021
N. E. Cusano (ed.), *Osteoporosis*,
https://doi.org/10.1007/978-3-030-83951-2_5

63

standing 5'6½" tall and weighing 129.4 pounds. There was no point tenderness or kyphoscoliosis of the spine. Rib-to-pelvis distance was three finger breadths bilaterally. Proximal muscle strength was intact with sit-to-stand and squatting. There was no anterior tibial tenderness, no fine resting tremor of outstretched hand, and no Cushingoid features.

She endorsed history of intermittent loose bowel movements alternating with constipation. Evaluation for secondary causes of osteoporosis (Table 5.1) showed an equivocally positive

Table 5.1 Results of biochemical evaluation

Test	Result	Reference
Calcium	9.5 mg/dL	8.6–10.0
Albumin	4.4 g/dL	3.4–4.8
Phosphate	4.6 mg/dL	2.7–4.5
Magnesium	2.2 mg	1.6–2.6
Creatinine	0.8 mg/dL	0.5–1.2
PTH	31.9 pg/mL	14–72
25OHD	43 ng/dL	25–80
Alkaline phosphatase	69 U/L	38–126
C-telopeptide	2188 pmol/L	Premenopausal <4500
BSAP	10 µg/L	Premenopausal ≤14
WBC	5.1 K/µL	4.5–11.0
Hemoglobin	14.1 g/dL	11.7–15.5
Platelet	349 K/µL	150–400
SPEP/UPEP immunofixation	No monoclonal protein	
Urine calcium	99 mg/24 h	100–250
Transglutaminase IgA antibody	27.9 U	<20
Iron	52 µg/dL	(50–170)
Total iron-binding capacity	462 µg/dL	(298–596)
Iron saturation	11%	(20–55)
Transferrin	310 mg/dL	(200–400)

25OHD 25-hydroxyvitamin D, *BSAP* bone-specific alkaline phosphatase, *WBC* white blood cell count, *SPEP/UPEP* serum and urine protein electrophoresis transglutaminase antibody level, prompting referral to gastroen-terology for upper gastrointestinal endoscopy. Microscopic evalu-ation biopsy samples from the second part of the duodenum showed diffuse mildly scalloped mucosa, chronic inflammation, increased intraepithelial lymphocytes, and partial villus blunting, findings consistent with celiac disease.

Assessment and Diagnosis

Many conditions, medications, and lifestyle factors may cause or contribute to osteoporosis (Table 5.2). Patients with densitometric osteoporosis, history of fragility fracture, low BMD Z-score, inci-dent fractures, or decreasing BMD on osteoporosis pharmacologic therapy should undergo evaluation for secondary causes of osteopo-rosis. Their identification may lead to alternative or adjunctive thera-pies and additional referral, or reconsideration of fracture risk estimates that may influence the decision to start, continue, or restart osteoporosis therapy. In subspecialty settings, secondary causes of osteoporosis have been found in 30% of cases in women [1], 60% in men [2], and 30% in patients presenting with fracture [3].

Often secondary causes of osteoporosis are asymptomatic and can only be discovered with laboratory testing. For assessment of secondary causes of osteoporosis in postmenopausal women, the American Association of Clinical Endocrinology recommends measurement of complete blood count, metabolic panel (includ-ing calcium, phosphate, total protein, albumin, creatinine, electro-lytes, AST, ALT, alkaline phosphatase), 25-hydroxyvitamin D, intact parathyroid hormone, and 24-h urine collection for calcium, sodium, and creatinine [4]. This battery of tests plus total testos-terone is recommended in the evaluation of male osteoporosis [5]. Additional tests if indicated may include TSH, transglutaminase antibody, serum protein electrophoresis and free light chains, uri-nary free cortisol, serum tryptase, bone marrow aspiration, tetracycline-labeled transilial bone biopsy, and genetic testing in suspected rare metabolic bone disease.

Selected contributors to bone loss are highlighted below. Vitamin D deficiency (whether defined as serum 25-hydroxyvitamin D <30

Table 5.2 Secondary causes of osteoporosis [4]

Endocrine or metabolic causes	Nutritional/GI conditions	Drugs	Genetic diseases	Others
Acromegaly	Alcoholism	Anti-epileptic drugs[a]	Ehlers Danlos syndrome	AIDS/HIV
Diabetes	Anorexia nervosa	Aromatase inhibitors	Familial dysautonomia	Ankylosing spondylitis
Type 1	Calcium deficiency	Chemotherapy	Gaucher disease	Hypercalciuria
Type 2	Chronic liver disease	Immunosuppressants	Glycogen storage diseases	Immobilization
Growth hormone deficiency	Malabsorption	Medroxyprogesterone	Homocystinuria	Major depression
Hypercortisolism	Syndromes/	Glucocorticoids	Marfan syndrome	Multiple myeloma monoclonal
Hyperparathyroidism	Malnutrition:	Gonadotropin-releasing hormone agents	Osteogenesis imperfecta	gammopathy of undetermined
Hyperprolactinemia	Celiac disease	Heparin		significance
Hyperthyroidism	Cystic fibrosis	Lithium		Organ transplantation
Hypogonadism	Crohn's disease	Proton pump inhibitors		Renal insufficiency
Hypophosphatasia	Gastric resection	Selective serotonin-reuptake inhibitors		Renal failure
Porphyria	Gastric bypass	sodium–glucose cotransporter-2 inhibitors		Renal tubular acidosis
Pregnancy	Total parenteral nutrition	Thiazolidinediones		Rheumatoid arthritis
	Vitamin D deficiency	Thyroid hormone (supraphysiologic doses)		Systemic mastocystosis
				Thalassemia

Adapted from American Association of Clinical Endocrinology Postmenopausal Osteoporosis Guidelines, 2020: Used with permission

[a]Phenobarbital, phenytoin, primidone, valproate, carbamazepine

or <20 ng/dL) may be due to inadequate solar exposure and vitamin D intake [6] and perhaps sequestration into adipose tissue and decreased bioavailability [7]. However, when coupled with elevated PTH, elevated alkaline phosphatase and bone pain (suggesting the presence of osteomalacia), vitamin D malabsorption should be considered. As vitamin D absorption occurs in the duodenum and proximal ileum, malabsorption in the setting of bariatric surgery and other small bowel pathologies may lead to vitamin D deficiency [8].

Secondary hyperparathyroidism is often a marker of calcium and/or vitamin D insufficiency and contributes to bone loss and increased risk for fracture. Whereas vitamin D status is readily assessed with a lab measurement of 25-hydroxyvitamin D, a 24-h urine collection may demonstrate calcium inadequacy. Low urinary calcium excretion of <50–100 mg/24 h suggests a need to address calcium supplementation, sometimes aggressively. Fractional calcium absorption decreases >70% in the setting of roux-en-Y gastric bypass even with maintenance of vitamin D sufficient status and good calcium intake [9]. This suggests that calcium supplementation greater [10] than general population recommendations (1000–1200 mg daily) [11] may be required to manage secondary hyperparathyroidism and calcium deficiency due to malabsorption [10].

Evaluation of secondary hyperparathyroidism with a 24-h urine collection may identify hypercalciuria, defined as a urinary calcium excretion of >300–350 mg/24 h [12]. Thiazide treatment, which improves calcium balance and reduces hyperparathyroidism, has been shown to improve bone density at the spine and hip in a clinical trial [13] and was associated with decreased hip fracture risk in an observational study [14].

Osteoporosis is a well-recognized result of systemic inflammation in disorders such as rheumatoid arthritis, Crohn's disease, and chronic obstructive pulmonary disease [15]. In such conditions, an active inflammatory milieu increases expression of RANKL, driving enhanced osteoclastogenesis, osteoclast activity, bone remodeling, and ultimately bone loss and deterioration. Additive contributors to fracture risk include glucocorticoid therapy, sedentary status, sarcopenia, and increased fall risk.

Multiple myeloma is the second most common hematologic malignancy and has the highest incidence of skeletal-related events among all malignant diseases [16]. In multiple myeloma, bone remodeling is uncoupled, characterized by enhanced osteoclastic activity and suppressed osteoblastic bone formation. The bone destructive process releases growth factors from the bone matrix, which contributes to further proliferation of multiple myeloma cells [17]. With uncoupled bone turnover, 15–20% of patients with newly diagnosed multiple myeloma present with hypercalcemia [17]. Anemia and renal insufficiency are also hallmarks of this disease, and this combination should lead to screening. Monoclonal gammopathy of uncertain significance (MGUS) is more common than MM and is also associated with greater risk of fracture especially of vertebrae versus control populations [18, 19].

Other endocrine diseases may be identified in the setting of osteoporosis such as hypogonadism, primary hyperparathyroidism, and thyrotoxicosis. Classic signs of Cushing's syndrome such as central obesity, "moon facies," striae, plethora, worsening diabetes, and hypertension point toward this diagnosis; however, more subtle findings of easy bruising, proximal muscle weakness, recurrent infections, or unexplained mood liability should prompt screening (dexamethasone suppression test, 24-h urinary free cortisol, or midnight salivary cortisol). Up to 50% of patients with hypercortisolism experience vertebral compression fractures [20]. Once Cushing's syndrome has been identified and treated, bone recovery can be slow, and patients benefit from concomitant treatment with osteoporosis therapy.

The prevalence of biopsy-proven celiac disease in an osteoporosis population was 1.6% among 3188 patients by meta-analysis [21]. In 400 patients with fracture of the distal radius or ankle, screening with transglutaminase IgA antibody led to new diagnosis of biopsy-proven celiac disease in 1.5% [22]. In 1042 patients attending a fracture liaison program, celiac disease was identified in 0.38% (4/1042) [23]. These data suggest against universal screening for celiac disease in an osteoporosis or fracture population. However, celiac disease in 693 patients enrolled in a BMD registry showed a higher risk for major osteoporotic fracture after FRAX adjustment, and inclusion of celiac disease as a secondary osteoporosis risk factor in FRAX approached the observed fracture risk [24]. This suggests the importance of a case-finding approach, and eliciting symptoms consistent with celiac disease should be followed by screening.

Outcome

For about 5 years prior to a diagnosis of celiac disease, the patient had already lowered dietary gluten intake, which may help explain "equivocal" baseline transglutaminase titers. In retrospect, she recalled transient erythematous rash (consistent with dermatitis herpetiformis) when she consumed small amounts of bread. She was instructed not to fill a prescription for oral bisphosphonate she was previously given, and lifestyle factors of gluten-free diet, calcium and vitamin D adequacy, and physical activity were

Table 5.3 Serial DXA BMD

	L1–L4 spine BMD (T-score) g/cm^2 change vs. prior; % change vs. prior	Left femoral neck BMD (T-score)	Left total hip BMD (T-score) g/cm^2 change vs. prior; % change vs. prior
2/22/2008	0.716 (−3.0)	0.638 (−1.9)	0.766 (−1.6)
2/23/2010	0.749 (−2.7) +0.033; +4.5%	0.680 (−1.5)	0.755 (−1.5) −0.011; −1.4%
2/29/2012	0.727 (−2.9) −0.022; −2.9%	0.649 (−1.8)	0.738 (−1.7) −0.017; −2.2%
3/11/2014	0.731 (−2.8) +0.004; +0.6%	0.665 (−1.7)	0.754 (−1.5) −0.016; +2.2%
5/3/2016	0.701 (−3.1) −0.030; −4.1%	0.689 (−1.4)	0.760 (−1.5) +0.006; +0.8%
5/2/2018	0.764 (−2.6) +0.063; +9.0%	0.680 (−1.5)	0.773 (−1.4) +0.013; +1.6%
5/21/2020	0.823 (−2.0) +0.059; +7.7%	0.681 (−1.5)	0.775 (−1.4) +0.002; +0.3%

Least significant change: 0.022 g/cm^2 at lumbar spine, 0.027 g/cm^2 at total hip emphasized. DXA scans were repeated every 2 years (Table 5.3). Based on this outside DXA facility's least significant change, BMD at the spine (and perhaps left femoral neck) improved from 2008 to 2010 and stabilized from 2010 to 2014; total hip BMD remained overall stable. However, spine BMD decreased from 2014 to 2016. In 2017, she started denosumab, followed by BMD improvements of 17.4% and 2.0% at the lumbar spine and left total hip, respectively, from 2016 to 2020, and she has remained fracture-free as of this writing. This case demonstrates the possibility of mild celiac disease presenting in a bone health clinic, without obvious gastrointestinal symptoms or signs such as iron-deficiency anemia.

References

1. Tannenbaum C, Clark J, Schwartzman K, et al. Yield of laboratory testing to identify secondary contributors to osteoporosis in otherwise healthy women. J Clin Endocrinol Metab. 2002;87(10):4431–7.
2. Kelepouris N, Harper KD, Gannon F, Kaplan FS, Haddad JG. Severe osteoporosis in men. Ann Intern Med. 1995;123(6):452–60.
3. Bogoch ER, Elliot-Gibson V, Wang RY, Josse RG. Secondary causes of osteoporosis in fracture patients. J Orthop Trauma. 2012;26(9):e145–52.
4. Camacho PM, Petak SM, Binkley N, et al. American Association of Clinical Endocrinologists/American College of Endocrinology Clinical Practice Guidelines for the diagnosis and treatment of postmenopausal osteoporosis-2020 update. Endocr Pract. 2020;26(Suppl 1):1–46.
5. Watts NB, Adler RA, Bilezikian JP, et al. Osteoporosis in men: an Endocrine Society clinical practice guideline. J Clin Endocrinol Metab. 2012;97(6):1802–22.
6. Dawson-Hughes B, Mithal A, Bonjour JP, et al. IOF position statement: vitamin D recommendations for older adults. Osteoporos Int. 2010;21(7):1151–4.
7. Migliaccio S, Di Nisio A, Mele C, et al. Obesity and hypovitaminosis D: causality or casualty? Int J Obes Suppl. 2019;9(1):20–31.
8. Johnson JM, Maher JW, DeMaria EJ, Downs RW, Wolfe LG, Kellum JM. The long-term effects of gastric bypass on vitamin D metabolism. Ann Surg. 2006;243(5):701–4; discussion 704–705.
9. Schafer AL, Weaver CM, Black DM, et al. Intestinal calcium absorption decreases dramatically after gastric bypass surgery despite optimization of vitamin D status. J Bone Miner Res. 2015;30(8):1377–85.
10. Flores L, Osaba MJM, Andreu A, Moize V, Rodriguez L, Vidal J. Calcium and vitamin D supplementation after gastric bypass should be individual-

ized to improve or avoid hyperparathyroidism. Obes Surg. 2010;20(6):738–43.

11. Ross AC, Manson JE, Abrams SA, et al. The 2011 report on dietary reference intakes for calcium and vitamin D from the Institute of Medicine: what clinicians need to know. J Clin Endocrinol Metab. 2011;96(1):53–8.

12. Ryan LE, Ing SW. Idiopathic hypercalciuria and bone health. Curr Osteoporos Rep. 2012;10(4):286–95.

13. LaCroix AZ, Ott SM, Ichikawa L, Scholes D, Barlow WE. Low-dose hydrochlorothiazide and preservation of bone mineral density in older adults. A randomized, double-blind, placebo-controlled trial. Ann Intern Med. 2000;133(7):516–26.

14. Feskanich D, Willett WC, Stampfer MJ, Colditz GA. A prospective study of thiazide use and fractures in women. Osteoporos Int. 1997;7(1):79–84.

15. Gravallese EM, Goldring S. Inflammation-induced bone loss in the rheumatic diseases. In: Bilezikian JP, editor. Primer on the metabolic bone diseases and disorders of mineral metabolism. 9th ed. Hoboken: Wiley-Blackwell; 2019. p. 459–66.

16. Siegel RL, Miller KD, Jemal A. Cancer statistics, 2020. CA Cancer J Clin. 2020;70(1):7–30.

17. O'Donnell EK, Raje NS. Myeloma bone disease: pathogenesis and treatment. Clin Adv Hematol Oncol. 2017;15(4):285–95.

18. Lomas OC, Mouhieddine TH, Tahri S, Ghobrial IM. Monoclonal gammopathy of undetermined significance (MGUS): not so asymptomatic after all. Cancers. 2020;12(6):1554.

19. Veronese N, Luchini C, Solmi M, Sergi G, Manzato E, Stubbs B. Monoclonal gammopathy of undetermined significance and bone health outcomes: a systematic review and exploratory meta-analysis. J Bone Miner Metab. 2018;36(1):128–32.

20. Vestergaard P, Lindholm J, Jorgensen JO, et al. Increased risk of osteoporotic fractures in patients with Cushing's syndrome. Eur J Endocrinol. 2002;146(1):51–6.

21. Laszkowska M, Mahadev S, Sundstrom J, et al. Systematic review with meta-analysis: the prevalence of coeliac disease in patients with osteoporosis. Aliment Pharmacol Ther. 2018;48(6):590–7.

22. Hjelle AM, Apalset E, Mielnik P, Nilsen RM, Lundin KEA, Tell GS. Positive IgA against transglutaminase 2 in patients with distal radius and ankle fractures compared to community-based controls. Scand J Gastroenterol. 2018;53(10–11):1212–6.

23. de Bruin IJA, Vranken L, Wyers CE, et al. The prevalence of celiac disease in a fracture liaison service population. Calcif Tissue Int. 2020;107(4):327–34.

24. Duerksen DR, Lix LM, Johansson H, et al. Fracture risk assessment in celiac disease: a registry-based cohort study. Osteoporos Int. 2021;32(1):93–9.

Osteoporosis in Premenopausal Women

Bente L. Langdahl

Case Presentation

A 36-year-old woman was diagnosed with ulcerative colitis at the age of 15. She was treated with different immunosuppressants: azathioprine, mesalazine, infliximab, and intermittently with oral glucocorticoids for many years. At the age of 23, colectomy was performed, and treatment with oral glucocorticoids was almost completely replaced by local treatment until the rectum was removed a year later. Supplementation with calcium and vitamin D was not given during the years with high doses of oral glucocorticoids.

Bone density testing was performed at the age of 27. BMD T-scores of the spine and hip were −2.7 and −3.3. The patient initiated treatment with alendronate, which worsened ulcerative colitis symptoms and alendronate was discontinued. The patient was considering pregnancy and treatment of osteoporosis apart from calcium and vitamin D supplementation was therefore not pursued further.

The patient was referred to our department for treatment of osteoporosis at age 30.

B. L. Langdahl (✉)
Department of Endocrinology and Internal Medicine, Aarhus University Hospital, Aarhus, Denmark
e-mail: bente.langdahl@aarhus.rm.dk

© The Author(s), under exclusive license to Springer Nature Switzerland AG 2021
N. E. Cusano (ed.), *Osteoporosis*,
https://doi.org/10.1007/978-3-030-83951-2_6

The patient stated she had regular menstrual periods, had not experienced any fractures with the exception of a forearm fracture as a child, and had no family history of osteoporosis or frequent fractures. She does not smoke and consumes less than 1 unit of alcohol per day. BMI was 22.2 kg/cm².

Laboratory evaluation was without signs of secondary osteoporosis. Genetic screening for osteogenesis imperfecta was not performed since the patient had only suffered a single fracture during childhood after a relevant trauma. BMD T-scores were −3.0 at the lumbar spine and −2.9 at the total hip. X-rays of the thoracic and lumbar spine demonstrated multiple vertebral fractures: T6 (40% loss of height), T8 (29%), T9 (28%), T10 (30%), T11 (24%), T12 (43%), L2 (38%), L3 (27%), and L4 (33%).

Assessment and Diagnosis

The fracture rate in premenopausal women is uncertain, but rare. The prevalence of osteoporotic T-scores in premenopausal women varies from 0.5% to 50% depending on the populations studied, the definition of osteoporosis used, and the referral center involved [1–4].

Bone mineral density of premenopausal women depends primarily on bone accrual during childhood and adolescence. Although 40–80% of the variation in BMD and bone microarchitecture is genetically determined [5], other factors including muscle mass, sexual development, and lifestyle factors, including calcium and vitamin D intake and physical activity, are also important [6]. The effect of most contraceptives on bone is neutral; however, the use of depot medroxyprogesterone acetate is associated with an increased risk of fracture [3].

For postmenopausal women, the diagnosis of osteoporosis is based on the World Health Organization operational definition, a BMD T-score ≤−2.5. For women between 20 and 40 years, the International Osteoporosis Foundation (IOF) recommends using the same definition as in post-menopausal women [2], whereas the International Society for Clinical Densitometry (ISCD) proposes using BMD Z-scores ≤-2 to define "bone density below the expected range for age" [7]. Vertebral or other major fragility fractures are considered a hallmark of osteoporosis by both societies. Idiopathic osteoporosis is defined as the occurrence of a low trauma fracture in the presence of low BMD (lumbar spine and or hip T score ≤-2.5 or Z-score ≤-2) after excluding causes of secondary osteoporosis [1, 3].

Osteoporosis in premenopausal women is often secondary to diseases, medical treatments, or lifestyle factors, including endocrine, inflammatory, neuromuscular, oncologic, hematologic, pulmonary, and gastrointestinal disorders and therapies, in addition to tobacco and alcohol use. Obtaining a thorough medical history and performing a biochemical evaluation are needed to exclude causes of secondary osteoporosis [1, 3]. In addition, screening for genetic causes is recommended when there is a strong suspicion of a heritable component based on family history and/or additional clinical features (syndromes) suggestive of underlying monogenetic bone disorders, such as osteogenesis imperfecta, hypophosphatasia, or osteoporosis-pseudoglioma syndrome [2].

There are special cases that need further consideration. Patients with anorexia nervosa, which in addition to low body weight is characterized by significant hormonal changes, including hypogonadism/other causes of amenorrhea, hypercortisolism, low testosterone, and low IGF-1 levels, often have low bone mass and sometimes suffer fractures [8]. Premenopausal women on diets excluding animal meat protein (vegetarianism) or any animal products (veganism) have in some studies been found to have an increased risk of fracture [9]. In premenopausal women with breast cancer, adjuvant therapy including chemotherapy and gonadotropin hormone-releasing hormone (GnRH) analogs can induce secondary amenorrhea and premature menopause. Moreover, treatment with tamoxifen, a selective estrogen receptor modulator which has antiestrogen effects in premenopausal women, has been associated with increased risk of fracture. Treatment with GnRH receptor antagonists for endometriosis is also associated with BMD loss [3]. Glucocorticoid-induced osteoporosis in premenopausal women is usually seen in patients with autoimmune or inflammatory disorders that may themselves cause osteoporosis. Glucocorticoids exert multiple negative effects on bone, but they also mitigate the negative effects of the underlying disease on bone health, and therefore it is the balance between these effects in combination with the dose and duration of the treatment that determines the outcome [10].

Pregnancy and lactation-associated osteoporosis (PLAO) [11] is a rare condition associated with changes in calcium metabolism occurring during pregnancy and lactation that lead to a transient bone loss, mainly at trabecular sites. Among the factors involved are parathyroid hormone-related protein and the need for additional calcium for mineralization of the fetal skeleton and the production of milk during lactation. In addition, studies have suggested that women developing PLAO may have an underlying osteoblast insufficiency. After lactation, bone mass and strength normally recover.

Hypovitaminosis D may lead to osteomalacia which should be differentiated from osteoporosis as this represents a mineralization deficit that in most cases is reversible. Low bone mass most often improves dramatically upon normalization of vitamin D.

Management

Once a diagnosis of osteoporosis has been made, the next step is to evaluate future fracture risk. Although classical risk factors should be considered, it is important to note that the FRAX® algorithm is not validated for individuals younger than 40 years. Premenopausal women with recent major fragility fractures are generally at high risk for further fractures in the short to medium term, but the risk depends on whether the condition is secondary to another condition that can be treated (e.g., celiac disease) or not.

Management of premenopausal osteoporosis is challenging due to a lack of robust evidence. There is some evidence that increases in calcium and vitamin D intake as well as physical activity may improve or stabilize BMD. In addition, cessation of smoking and excess alcohol consumption is generally recommended [1, 3].

Antiresorptive and bone forming treatments improve BMD in premenopausal women with idiopathic or secondary osteoporosis; however, fracture risk reduction has not been demonstrated (reviewed in [1–3]).

In patients with anorexia nervosa, weight gain and reappearance of regular menstrual periods are important determinants for the recovery of BMD [12].

For premenopausal women treated with glucocorticoids, the current guidelines are not in complete agreement. The joint IOF and ECTS guidelines recommend treatment in premenopausal woman with a previous fragility fracture taking oral glucocorticoid for at least 3 months, while for women without fracture, the treatment decision should be based on clinical judgment [13]. The American College of Rheumatology guidelines recommend treatment with oral bisphosphonates in premenopausal women treated with glucocorticoids at a daily dose ≥ 7.5 mg for ≥ 6 months in the presence of a fragility fracture or BMD Z-score <-3 [14].

In premenopausal women with breast cancer and hormone ablation therapy, it has been suggested that bisphosphonates should be initiated in women with a Z score <-2. In women with a Z score ≤ -1 and a 5–10% annual decrease in BMD, bisphosphonates are also suggested [3].

Cessation of lactation in women with PLAO leads to increases in BMD. Women treated with a bisphosphonate or teriparatide experienced larger increases in BMD compared to untreated women; however, none of these studies were powered to investigate the effect on fracture risk [11].

The risk of adverse effects should be considered as part of making treatment decisions for an individual patient. In addition to considering the usual adverse effects, the risk of potential teratogenic effects of the drug during a pregnancy should be considered. The majority of the literature regarding bisphosphonate use in humans does not report severe adverse fetal or maternal events; however, there are reports of spontaneous abortions [3]. As a measure of safety, it has been proposed that bisphosphonate treatment should not be initiated if a woman is planning a pregnancy within the next 12 months. Due to the lack of studies in pregnant women, denosumab and teriparatide are contraindicated in pregnancy.

Outcome

Treatment options including teriparatide and bisphosphonates were discussed with the patient. The patient decided that she wanted to have children and therefore no treatment was initiated. In September 2015, the patient gave birth to a daughter. In November 2015, 2 months after delivery, the patient complained of back pain. The patient was still breastfeeding the baby. DXA showed relatively stable BMD with T-scores at the spine and hip of −2.8 and −2.8, respectively. No X-ray was performed as the back pain was ascribed to the existing vertebral fractures. In March 2017, the patient again had symptoms of intermittent back pain. BMD T-scores of the spine and hip were −2.4 and −2.8, respectively. The patient was planning a second pregnancy, and treatment was therefore not initiated. In August 2018, the patient gave birth to twin sons. In November 2018, the patient came to the outpatient clinic and complained of acute severe low back pain, and X-ray of the spine showed a new compression fracture of L5.

The patient stopped breastfeeding in order to start anti-osteoporosis treatment. Due to the expected catabolic bone status due to pregnancy and lactation, treatment with zoledronic acid was given in December 2018. In March 2019, BMD T-scores were −2.7 and −2.9, respectively, which represented a significant BMD loss at the lumbar spine. Treatment with teriparatide was initiated.

In August 2019, 6 months after initiating teriparatide, the patient was still having severe back pain. Continuing pain many months after a vertebral fracture should always lead to reflection and further investigation as clinically indicated. New fractures, worsening of existing fractures, or other causes of back pain should be considered and investigated. MRI of the spine was performed and showed no new fractures or other pathologies. Edema was seen in L5, suggesting that the L5 fracture was not completely healed, whereas the older fractures were. There is no evidence that vertebroplasty reduces pain due to spine fractures better than medical treatment; however, we had tried medical treatment in combination with physiotherapy for 6 months with only minor improvement in pain. Vertebroplasty of L5 was performed with modest effect on the pain.

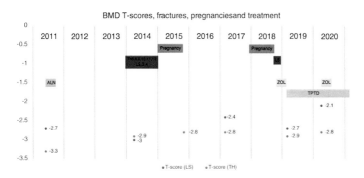

Fig. 6.1 The results of DXA performed over the years in the case are presented. In addition, the two pregnancies (orange boxes), vertebral fractures seen on X-rays (red boxes), and treatments: alendronate (ALN) (green box), zoledronate (ZOL) (yellow boxes), and teriparatide (TPTD) (blue box) are displayed

In April 2020, DXA showed increases in BMD at the spine and hip of 9.1% and 2.2%, respectively. Treatment with teriparatide continues, and the patient had a second infusion of zoledronate in May 2020 because BMD of the hip was still very low and bone loss at the hip should be avoided (see Fig. 6.1 for overview).

Severe osteoporosis with multiple vertebral fractures, back pain, and inability to take care of her three young children due to her disability has been a very difficult situation for the whole family. Despite getting help with household and childcare issues, the patient's husband has been on sick leave due to stress. In addition, the patient had tried working again as a laboratory technician after her maternity leave, but she was not able to work and is now permanently retired. Severe osteoporosis does not only affect the patient, but the entire family, especially when this includes three young children, so we have to include the whole family in the management of the disease.

We have no measurement of BMD before this patient started glucocorticoid treatment as a teenager, but it is a reasonable assumption that the many years of glucocorticoid treatment without calcium and vitamin D supplementation played an important role in the development of severe osteoporosis in this premenopausal woman. It is unlikely that patients now would be treated for many years with glucocorticoids without supplementation with calcium and vitamin and without having DXA performed to monitor bone health. It cannot be determined if the pregnancies and the changes in calcium metabolism associated with pregnancy and lactation were the cause of the new vertebral fracture, but the occurrence of the fracture 3 months after delivery of her twin sons would fit with what is often seen in PLAO and with the notion that PLAO more often occurs in women with preexisting low bone mass or poor bone quality.

This case demonstrates that osteoporosis in premenopausal women is less straightforward than in postmenopausal women. The diagnosis is delayed because osteoporosis is rare in premenopausal women and therefore often not considered even in the presence of conditions or pharmacologic treatments known to be associated with risk of osteoporosis. Although there is increasing evidence of the beneficial effect of antiresorptive and bone-forming treatments on bone turnover and BMD in premenopausal women, there is no evidence for anti-fracture efficacy. The treatment plan has to take family planning into account as therapy should not be used in pregnant women and women planning pregnancy. This in combination with the temporary loss of BMD during pregnancy and lactation makes treatment of osteoporosis in premenopausal women a task for specialists.

Clinical Pearls/Pitfalls
- Osteoporosis in premenopausal women is often secondary to other diseases and pharmacologic treatments, most frequently diseases that involve inflammation and glucocorticoid treatment. Correction or treatment of the secondary cause should be considered if at all possible.
- Once a diagnosis of premenopausal osteoporosis is made using BMD T-score ≤ -2.5 or Z-score ≤ -2 and a major fragility fracture, the patient should be referred to an osteoporosis specialist for treatment.

- The increased risk of osteoporosis associated with a number of diseases and treatments in premenopausal women should be included in relevant guidelines, and physicians should be aware of this complication in order to avoid delay of diagnosis.
- Pregnancy and lactation-associated osteoporosis is a rare condition but gynecologists and obstetricians should keep this in mind in women with severe back pain during the last trimester or in the months following delivery.

References

1. Langdahl BL. Osteoporosis in premenopausal women. Curr Opin Rheumatol. 2017;29(4):410–5.
2. Ferrari S, Bianchi ML, Eisman JA, Foldes AJ, Adami S, Wahl DA, et al. Osteoporosis in young adults: pathophysiology, diagnosis, and management. Osteoporos Int. 2012;23(12):2735–48.
3. Pepe J, Body JJ, Hadji P, McCloskey E, Meier C, Obermayer-Pietsch B, et al. Osteoporosis in premenopausal women: a clinical narrative review by the ECTS and the IOF. J Clin Endocrinol Metab. 2020;105(8):dgaa306.
4. Cohen A. Premenopausal osteoporosis. Endocrinol Metab Clin N Am. 2017;46(1):117–33.
5. Gordon CM, Zemel BS, Wren TA, Leonard MB, Bachrach LK, Rauch F, et al. The determinants of peak bone mass. J Pediatr. 2017;180:261–9.
6. Weaver CM, Gordon CM, Janz KF, Kalkwarf HJ, Lappe JM, Lewis R, et al. The National Osteoporosis Foundation's position statement on peak bone mass development and lifestyle factors: a systematic review and implementation recommendations. Osteoporos Int. 2016;27(4):1281–386.
7. Lewiecki EM, Gordon CM, Baim S, Binkley N, Bilezikian JP, Kendler DL, et al. Special report on the 2007 adult and pediatric Position Development Conferences of the International Society for Clinical Densitometry. Osteoporos Int. 2008;19(10):1369–78.
8. Solmi M, Veronese N, Correll CU, Favaro A, Santonastaso P, Caregaro L, et al. Bone mineral density, osteoporosis, and fractures among people with eating disorders: a systematic review and meta-analysis. Acta Psychiatr Scand. 2016;133(5):341–51.
9. Ho-Pham LT, Nguyen ND, Nguyen TV. Effect of vegetarian diets on bone mineral density: a Bayesian meta-analysis. Am J Clin Nutr. 2009;90(4):943–50.

10. Buckley L, Humphrey MB. Glucocorticoid-induced osteoporosis. N Engl J Med. 2018;379(26):2547–56.
11. Kovacs CS, Ralston SH. Presentation and management of osteoporosis presenting in association with pregnancy or lactation. Osteoporos Int. 2015;26(9):2223–41.
12. Miller KK, Lee EE, Lawson EA, Misra M, Minihan J, Grinspoon SK, et al. Determinants of skeletal loss and recovery in anorexia nervosa. J Clin Endocrinol Metab. 2006;91(8):2931–7.
13. Lekamwasam S, Adachi JD, Agnusdei D, Bilezikian J, Boonen S, Borgstrom F, et al. A framework for the development of guidelines for the management of glucocorticoid-induced osteoporosis. Osteoporos Int. 2012;23(9):2257–76.
14. Buckley L, Guyatt G, Fink HA, Cannon M, Grossman J, Hansen KE, et al. 2017 American College of Rheumatology Guideline for the prevention and treatment of glucocorticoid-induced osteoporosis. Arthritis Rheumatol. 2017;69(8):1521–37.

Osteoporosis in Men

7

Brinda Manchireddy,
Maria Gabriela Negron Marte,
and Robert A. Adler

Case

A 58-year-old Caucasian man with a past history of degenerative disc disease, osteoarthritis, severe gastroesophageal reflux disease (GERD), alcohol dependence, hepatic steatosis, and prior heavy smoking was initially referred for evaluation for osteoporosis after presenting to the emergency department with complaints of back pain. He was found to have compression deformities of T4–T7 with evidence of an acute compression fracture of T7. He reported significant loss of height but no history of trauma. Upon further interview, it was noted he had a T4 compression fracture at age 53 that was evident on an X-ray, which led to bone mineral density testing but no treatment. He underwent a kyphoplasty at T7 before our evaluation.

The patient had no family history of osteoporosis or prior use of glucocorticoids or androgen deprivation therapy. He did not consume dairy products or eat other calcium rich foods but reported taking cholecalciferol 2000 international units (50 μg)

B. Manchireddy · M. G. N. Marte · R. A. Adler (✉)
Endocrinology and Metabolism Section, Central Virginia Veterans
Affairs Health Care System and Division of Endocrinology, Metabolism,
and Diabetes, Virginia Commonwealth University, Richmond, VA, USA
e-mail: mariagabriela.negronmarte@vcuhealth.org; Robert.adler@va.gov

daily. His physical activity was limited by back pain. On exam, he was in a wheelchair because of the distance from the parking lot to the clinic. Vital signs were normal, and his BMI was 32.5 kg/m². Height measurements had not been taken previously; the patient had provided his estimated height. He had a few teeth in poor condition, and his back was diffusely tender to palpation.

Assessment and Diagnosis

Basic laboratory tests were normal: calcium, phosphate, albumin, renal function, and alkaline phosphatase. His 25-hydroxyvitamin D level was 25.4 ng/mL. A spot urine calcium to creatinine ratio was low. Given the patient's young age, additional laboratories were obtained to exclude secondary causes such as hypogonadism and hyperthyroidism. Malabsorption and celiac disease were not assessed. One year prior to presentation, a bone mineral density demonstrated borderline osteopenia with T-scores of -1 at both the lumbar spine and hip. His atraumatic fractures of the spine were enough to justify the diagnosis of osteoporosis and to require treatment.

Osteoporosis is a musculoskeletal disease characterized by decreased bone quantity as measured by bone mineral density and decreased bone quality, resulting in increased risk of fragility fractures. For a long time, men were not screened for osteoporosis until further investigation revealed the impact of fractures in men on morbidity, mortality, and societal cost.

According to the WHO diagnostic classification, osteoporosis is defined by BMD at the hip or lumbar spine that is less than or equal to 2.5 standard deviations below the mean BMD of a young-adult reference population. This is expressed as a T-score of −2.5. Most organizations believe that the young adult white female database should be used for the calculation of the T-score for all adults. Low bone mass or osteopenia is defined as a T-score between −1 and −2.5, and the great majority of fractures occur in such people because there are so many more people in this category. However, it is instructive to note that fragility fractures can occur in some patients with normal bone density, suggesting that poor bone quality is the reason for their fracture risk, as illustrated by this case. The Endocrine Society Male Osteoporosis Guideline [1] suggests that men should be screened for osteoporosis with BMD at age 70. A recent observational study [2] reported that performing BMD testing at age 80 led to fewer fractures.

Trabecular bone score (TBS) is a recently developed tool that performs novel gray-level texture analysis on lumbar spine DXA images and thereby captures information relating to trabecular microarchitecture, a possible indicator of bone quality. For TBS to usefully add to BMD and clinical risk factors in osteoporosis risk stratification, it must be independently associated with fracture risk, readily obtainable, and, ideally, present a risk which is amenable to osteoporosis treatment [3].

There are two main types of osteoporosis in men: primary and secondary. In cases of primary osteoporosis, either the condition is caused by age-related bone loss (sometimes called *senile osteoporosis*) or the cause is unknown (*idiopathic osteoporosis*). The term idiopathic osteoporosis is typically used only for men younger than 70 years old; in older men, age-related bone loss is assumed to be the cause, although there may be many risk factors present [4–6]. There are multiple theories as to the etiology of idiopathic male osteoporosis, such as genetic factors or a family history. Several epidemiological and clinical observations have shown that osteoporosis in both men and women has an important genetic component. Multiple genes may have effects on bone development, strength, and density [7]. In many studies, most men with osteoporosis have at least one (sometimes more than one) secondary cause. In cases of secondary osteoporosis, low bone mass is due to certain lifestyle behaviors, diseases, or medications [4–6].

Secondary causes in men include the use of glucocorticoids, immunosuppressive drugs, hypogonadism, excessive alcohol consumption, smoking, chronic obstructive pulmonary disease (COPD) or asthma, cystic fibrosis, malabsorption, hypercalciuria, anticonvulsant medications, thyrotoxicosis, hyperparathyroidism, immobilization, bariatric surgery, ankylosing spondylitis, rheumatoid arthritis, and systemic mastocytosis. There is overlap between what could be called a risk factor for osteoporosis and a secondary cause [5, 6]. Of the listed secondary causes, medications (especially glucocorticoids, androgen deprivation therapy for prostate cancer, and anti-seizure medications), COPD, hyper-parathyroidism, alcohol abuse, hypercalciuria, and hypogonadism are probably the most common causes of secondary osteoporosis in men.

Management

Risks and benefits of osteoporosis treatment were discussed with the patient after which he elected to start therapy with intravenous zoledronic acid. He was not a good candidate for daily injections of the anabolic agent teriparatide because of his alcohol abuse, and he had severe gastroesophageal reflux disease, which made oral bisphosphonates not a good choice. The patient subsequently received three doses of zoledronic acid over 4 years. In addition, he was counseled on fall prevention strategies, advised to perform weight-bearing exercises, and recommended to consume 1200 mg of calcium and 2000 IU of vitamin D daily.

The patient was seen annually in the metabolic bone clinic, and his vitamin D supplementation was adjusted to a target of 25-hydroxyvitmain D >30 ng/mL. He was ambulating with a cane and had incorporated dairy into his diet (yogurt and cheese). Physical exam during follow-up visits was notable for obesity, mild kyphosis, and poor dentition (but no osteonecrosis of the jaw). A follow-up BMD demonstrated increased density in the spine and total hip, 4.9% and 2.3%, respectively (see Table 7.1). However, the spine trabecular bone score (TBS) T-score was

Table 7.1 Comparison between pretreatment (initial) and posttreatment (after 3.5 years) BMD

BMD	T-score spine L1–4	T-score right hip	T-score femoral neck	T-score distal 1/3 radius
Pretreatment (08/2014)	−1	+0.7	−1	+1.5
Posttreatment (02/2019)	−0.2	1.8	−0.8	+2.7

−2.3; it had not been available previously. A full-length image of his left femur did not show any early evidence of atypical fracture.

Age-appropriate intake of calcium and vitamin D is advised for all patients. The National Academy of Medicine (formerly the Institute of Medicine) recommends men ages 50–70 consume 1000 mg/day of elemental calcium [8]. If an adequate dietary intake cannot be achieved, calcium supplements should be used. For adults age 50 and older, a vitamin D intake of 800–1000 IU daily is recommended by the National Osteoporosis Foundation [9].

As with our patient, and with any patient at risk of deficiency or with osteoporosis, 25-hydroxyvitamin D levels should be measured. Supplements should be recommended with the goal of achieving a serum 25-hydroxyvitamin D level of approximately 30 ng/mL [10]. While vitamin D deficiency can be treated with weekly doses of ergocalciferol at 50,000 IU/week for 8–12 weeks, many experts prefer cholecalciferol in daily doses of up to 4000 IU (100 μg) daily with lower doses as maintenance.

Regular weight-bearing and muscle-strengthening exercises are recommended with the intention of improving agility, strength, and balance. Some examples are Tai Chi, walking, jogging, tennis, and weight training. Fall risk assessment should be individualized and will be impacted by all the above. Other potentially modifiable factors include vision impairment, polypharmacy, and home safety. Tobacco use cessation and avoidance of excessive alcohol consumption are also crucial parts of this comprehensive approach to osteoporosis management.

The US FDA-approved pharmacotherapy for osteoporosis treatment in men includes bisphosphonates (alendronate, risedronate, ibandronate, and zoledronic acid), teriparatide, and denosumab. Among bisphosphonates, zoledronic acid increased bone density to a greater extent in men on oral glucocorticoids than did risedronate [11]. In an international trial with vertebral fracture as the primary outcome, intravenous zoledronic acid was found to provide a 67% relative fracture risk reduction, compared to placebo infusion [12]. This is similar to the drug's impact in women.

Denosumab was initially approved in 2011 to increase bone mass in men at high risk for fracture receiving androgen deprivation therapy for nonmetastatic prostate cancer. The following year, it was approved to increase bone mass in men with osteoporosis at high risk for fracture or those who have failed or are intolerant to other therapies [13].

The anabolic agent teriparatide is indicated for treatment of male osteoporosis with high fracture risk and for glucocorticoid-induced osteoporosis. It has shown equivalent increases in BMD in men and women; interestingly, the described bone loss after discontinuation of therapy was greater in women than men [14].

Abaloparatide is a modification of parathyroid hormone-related peptide approved for treatment of osteoporosis in postmenopausal women. Recent studies [15, 16] have shown that in osteopenic orchiectomized rats, abaloparatide can increase endocortical bone formation and improve trabecular bone volume and microarchitecture by augmenting osteoblast numbers without increasing osteoclast numbers. Based on the above, it may be warranted to consider off-label use of this drug for male osteoporosis. There is an ongoing study of abaloparatide in men with osteoporosis. The newest anabolic agent, romosozumab, is FDA approved for postmenopausal women, but there is evidence [17] that it works similarly in men.

It is worth mentioning that treatment decisions are made according to the patient's comorbidities, preferences, and cost. In clinical practice, it is common to have patients start on antiresorptive therapy (usually oral bisphosphonates) and later transition to anabolic agents after intolerance, unsatisfactory response, or drug failure. However, prior use of bisphosphonates may blunt or delay the impact of anabolic agents on bone density [18, 19]. For this reason, many experts now suggest using anabolic drugs first in patients at highest risk for fracture. There are no studies of drug holidays or even long-term treatment of osteoporosis in men. Hence, general recommendations for women (e.g., [20]) are used to guide long-term treatment.

Outcome

At the most recent visit, which was by telephone because of the pandemic, the patient had been sober for 2 years, had stayed off tobacco, and had improved his diet and exercise. A follow-up in person assessment and repeat BMD were planned to consider whether anabolic treatment or other anti-resorptive therapy would be helpful at this time. He has had no further clinical fractures.

Clinical Pearls
- Osteoporosis needs to be evaluated and treated in men.
- Fractures can occur in patients with normal bone density. A clinical fracture is a sentinel event.
- Evaluation and treatment of men are similar to that in women.
- Very high fracture risk patients should be considered for anabolic treatment first.

Conflict of Interest: Drs. Manchireddy and Negron Marte have no conflicts of interest. Dr. Adler was site principal investigator of a study of abalaparatide sponsored by the manufacturer. All funds went to the institution.

References

1. Watts NB, et al. Osteoporosis in men: an Endocrine Society clinical practice guideline. J Clin Endocrinol Metab. 2012;97(6):1802–22.
2. Colon-Emeric CS, et al. Limited osteoporosis screening effectiveness due to low treatment rates in a national sample of older men. Mayo Clin Proc. 2018;93:1749–59.
3. Harvey NC, et al. Trabecular bone score (TBS) as a new complementary approach for osteoporosis evaluation in clinical practice. Bone. 2015;78:216–24.
4. Willson T, et al. The clinical epidemiology of male osteoporosis: a review of the recent literature. Clin Epidemiol. 2015;7:65–76.
5. Adler RA. Update on osteoporosis in men. Best Pract Res Clin Endocrinol Metab. 2018;32:758–72.
6. Ryan CS, et al. Osteoporosis in men: the value of laboratory testing. Osteoporos Int. 2011;22:1845–53.
7. Chen S, et al. Genetic burden contributing to extremely high or low bone mineral density in a senior male population from the osteoporotic fractures in men study (MrOS). JBMR Plus. 2020;4(3):e10335.

8. Ross AC, et al. The 2011 report on dietary reference intakes for calcium and vitamin D from the Institute of Medicine: what clinicians need to know. J Clin Endocrinol Metab. 2011;96(1):53–8.

9. Cosman F, et al. Clinician's guide to prevention and treatment of osteoporosis. Osteoporos Int. 2014;25(10):2359–81.

10. El-Hajj Fuleihan G, et al. Serum 25-hydroxyvitamin D levels: variability, knowledge gaps, and the concept of a desirable range. J Bone Miner Res. 2015;30:1119–33.

11. Reid DM, et al. Zoledronic acid and risedronate in the prevention and treatment of glucocorticoid-induced osteoporosis (HORIZON): a multi-centre, double-blind, double-dummy, randomized controlled trial. Lancet. 2009;373:1253–63.

12. Boonen S, et al. Fracture risk and zoledronic acid therapy in men with osteoporosis. N Engl J Med. 2012;367:1714–23.

13. Sidlauskas KM, et al. Osteoporosis in men: epidemiology and treatment with denosumab. Clin Interv Aging. 2014;9:593–601.

14. Leder BZ, et al. Effects of teriparatide treatment and discontinuation in postmenopausal women and eugonadal men with osteoporosis. J Clin Endocrinol Metab. 2009;94(8):2915–21.

15. Besschetnova T, et al. Abaloparatide improves cortical geometry and trabecular microarchitecture and increases vertebral and femoral neck strength in a rat model of male osteoporosis. Bone. 2019;124:148–57.

16. Chandler H, Lanske B, Aurore Varela A, et al. Abaloparatide, a novel osteoanabolic PTHrP analog, increases cortical and trabecular bone mass and architecture in orchiectomized rats by increasing bone formation without increasing bone resorption. Bone. 2019;120:148–55.

17. Lewiecki EM, et al. A phase III randomized placebo-controlled trial to evaluate efficacy and safety of romosozumab in men with osteoporosis. J Clin Endocrinol Metab. 2018;103:3183–93.

18. Leder BZ. Optimizing sequential and combined anabolic and antiresorptive osteoporosis therapy. JBMR Plus. 2018;2(2):62–8.

19. Cosman F. Anabolic therapy and optimal treatment sequences for patients with osteoporosis at high risk for fracture. Endocr Pract. 2020;26(7):777–86.

20. Adler RA, et al. Managing osteoporosis in patients on long-term bisphosphonate treatment: report of a task force of the American Society for Bone and Mineral Research. J Bone Miner Res. 2016;31(1):16–35.

Osteoporosis in the Elderly

8

Parinya Samakkarnthai and Jad G. Sfeir

Case Presentation

A 76-year-old woman, with a history of Alzheimer dementia (Functional Assessment Staging Tool (FAST) stage 7, advanced) and currently living in a memory care unit, is evaluated in the emergency department following a fall while ambulating to the bathroom after which she was unable to get up or bear weight. Her medical history includes hypertension, hypothyroidism, and urinary incontinence, but no previous fractures. She had been hospitalized 3 years ago following a fall in the bathtub at home, resulting in superficial bruises and pain but no fractures. At that

P. Samakkarnthai
Robert and Arlene Kogod Center on Aging, Mayo Clinic, Rochester, MN, USA

Division of Endocrinology, Phramongkutklao Hospital and College of Medicine, Bangkok, Thailand

J. G. Sfeir (✉)
Robert and Arlene Kogod Center on Aging, Mayo Clinic, Rochester, MN, USA

Division of Endocrinology, Diabetes, Metabolism, and Nutrition; Division of Geriatric Medicine and Gerontology, Mayo Clinic, Rochester, MN, USA
e-mail: Sfeir.Jad@mayo.edu

© The Author(s), under exclusive license to Springer Nature Switzerland AG 2021
N. E. Cusano (ed.), *Osteoporosis*,
https://doi.org/10.1007/978-3-030-83951-2_8

Table 8.1 Laboratory results of patient upon presentation

	Results	Reference range
Calcium	8.8 mg/dL	8.8–10.2 mg/dL
Creatinine	0.83 mg/dL	0.59–1.04 mg/dL
Sodium	144 mmol/L	135–145 mmol/L
TSH	8.1 mIU/L	0.3–4.2 mIU/L
Free T4	1.1 ng/dL	0.9–1.7 ng/dL
25OHD	7.8 ng/mL	20–50 ng/mL

time, bone mineral density (BMD) showed a lowest T-score of
−1.7 and her 10-year fracture risk using the FRAX calculator
demonstrated 12% risk for major osteoporotic fracture and 2.9%
for hip fracture. Her medications include levothyroxine 50 mcg
daily, quetiapine 25 mg at bedtime, escitalopram 10 mg daily, and
famotidine 20 mg twice a day. On examination, her weight is
61.6 kg (65.4 kg 3 years ago) with a BMI of 24.1 kg/m^2. Her left
lower extremity is notably shortened and externally rotated; significant tenderness is noted to minimal touch of the left hip.
Laboratory results are notable for hypovitaminosis D (Table 8.1).
A left hip X-ray (Fig. 8.1) reveals a comminuted and displaced
intertrochanteric fracture of the left proximal femur.

Assessment and Diagnosis

Evaluation of musculoskeletal health in the elderly carries particular complexity as it involves an interplay of numerous factors
that are not necessarily present in younger adults. Multi-morbidity,
polypharmacy, social and community resources, and physical and
cognitive dysfunction, all influence our approach to osteoporosis
in older adults.

The interactions between bone, muscle, and fat are even more
pronounced with age leading to osteosarcopenia and frailty.
Consequently, the assessment of bone health in the elderly is not
complete without evaluation of muscle mass and function.
Multiple tools are available to assess for sarcopenia, but many
have limited clinical availability or incur significant time and cost
[1]. BMI and body circumference are not considered reliable to
evaluate for sarcopenia. Gait speed or Timed Up and Go (TUG)

Fig. 8.1 X-ray of left femur showing an intertrochanteric fracture of the left proximal femur (arrow). Also seen are displaced greater trochanteric and lesser trochanteric fragments

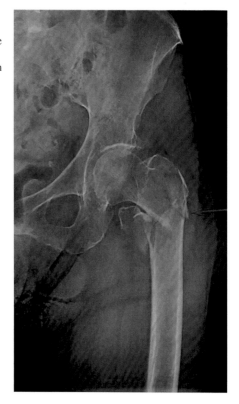

are easy tools to replicate in the clinic and can provide valuable physical performance assessment [2, 3]. Grip strength has been shown to have significant clinical relevance but requires a calibrated dynamometer and consistent measurement environment [4, 5]. Muscle mass assessment tools, on the other hand, are less readily available and provide limited clinical applicability at this time [1].

Fall risk evaluation can be achieved by short questionnaires. A prior history of falls, particularly in the past 12 months, is a significant risk factor for future falls [6]. A detailed evaluation of patients' living conditions, preferably performed on-site in their homes, adds significant insights into their health risks and barriers for improvement.

Polypharmacy (concomitant use of three or more medications), which impacts 67% of older adults, is known to be associated with a significant number of drug interactions and side effects. Medication use is one of the most modifiable risk factors for falls. Drugs that target the central nervous system, such as benzodiazepines and antidepressants, appear to be the most common drugs associated with falls [7, 8]. In addition, observational studies have reported increased risk of fractures among users of selective serotonin reuptake inhibitors (SSRIs) [9, 10].

Cognitive impairment is also associated with higher risks of falls and hip fractures. A meta-analysis found that cognitive impairment, specifically dysfunction in executive domains, was associated with falls [11].

Urinary incontinence is common in the elderly population and causes significant psychosocial stress. Further, it may lead to increased fall risk, particularly at nighttime. In multivariate analyses, incontinence was independently associated with risk of falling (OR 1.26; 95% CI 1.14–1.40) and with non-spine nontraumatic fractures (HR 1.34; 95% CI 1.06–1.69) [12]. Moreover, urinary incontinence may coexist with other autonomic dysfunction, further increasing the risk of falls. Thus, early detection and appropriate management of urinary incontinence, as well as associated sensory/autonomic dysfunction, are essential for fracture prevention.

The clinical assessment of osteoporosis in older adults is thus quite complex. Further complicating the issue is our inability to quantify all these risk factors that play an important role in mediating skeletal fragility. Commonly used fracture risk assessment tools (e.g., FRAX) do not fully account for frailty or sarcopenia and may thus underestimate the fracture risk in older adults [13]. The Fracture Risk Assessment in Long-term Care (FRAiL) calculator is a tool that relies on a host of clinical factors, including physical performance and muscle function, to predict the 2-year risk for hip fractures in adults residing in nursing homes [14]. Such approaches may prove more useful to derive comprehensive management plans in the elderly population.

Management

The management of osteoporosis and/or osteosarcopenia in older adults is also more intricate than that of younger patients. Care should be taken to recognize the cumulative burden of polypharmacy, barriers to compliance including cognitive function, presence and burden of comorbidities, living conditions and availability of community resources, as well as life and health expectancy of the individual patient. In addition to addressing underlying chronic illnesses that may be contributing to frailty and skeletal fragility, our goal is to reduce the risk of future falls and fractures while maintaining, or even improving, overall musculoskeletal health. It is thus important to discuss upfront the goals of care in order to generate a pragmatic and personalized management plan.

A good understanding of resources available to the patients at home and in their local communities will prove very important in the applicability of the management plan. Resources such as geriatric-friendly fitness centers, accessible transportation, nursing home visit programs, caretaker availability and health literacy, and affordable home modification strategies are essential to the success of our "osteoporosis prescription" in this population.

Nutrition plays a central role in such a management plan. An overall dietary plan, preferably by a nutrition specialist, should also be personalized. If sarcopenia is present, a protein-rich diet is advisable, despite lack of consensus on optimal protein content to maintain muscle mass in older adults.

Calcium and vitamin D are also vital for musculoskeletal health. There is evidence to suggest that men and women over age 65 years with low serum 25-hydroxyvitamin D concentrations (<10 ng/mL) are at greater risk for decreased muscle strength and increased hip fractures rates [15, 16]. Vitamin D supplementation may improve BMD and muscle function, particularly in patients with hypovitaminosis D [17]. The effect of vitamin D on risk of falls remains controversial but may be of particular importance in institutionalized older adults [18–20].

The National Academy of Medicine (formerly the Institute of Medicine) recommends 1200 mg of calcium per day and 800 IU of vitamin D per day in all adults 70 years or older. A higher vitamin D dose may be needed in those with established osteoporosis and/or sarcopenia. Assessing calcium and vitamin D intake from all sources can help in providing adequate recommendations for additional supplements. These include dietary sources of calcium (fish, milk, nuts, tofu) and vitamin D (oily fish, fortified juices, milk), sun exposure, as well as all multivitamins and supplements. A total daily calcium intake not exceeding 2000–2500 mg is considered safe by the National Osteoporosis Foundation and the American Society for Preventative Cardiology. Vitamin D doses up to 2000 IU per day are similarly very safe [20].

Exercise is one of the most consistent interventions to reduce the risk of falls [21, 22]. Exercise recommendations should aim at strengthening core muscles and improving balance in order to prevent subsequent falls. Resistance training, including weight-bearing and middle-to-high impact exercises, has been shown to improve bone health and BMD [23]. Any exercise program should build on the individual patient's baseline capacities and be progressively increased as tolerated to achieve a sustainable program [24, 25].

Pharmacologic interventions for fracture prevention parallel those for all adults with osteoporosis. Data from randomized trials, although limited by the small number of subjects beyond 75–80 years of age who were included in these studies, show continued effectiveness in older age. Risks for side effects associated with cumulative dosing of antiresorptive therapy may not be as important in those with lower life expectancy, resulting in a much more favorable risk-to-benefit balance.

The choice of pharmacologic agents should take into account the patient's neurobehavioral and social environments. For example, a parenteral medication given in a healthcare facility at regular intervals may be preferred over an oral weekly medication in patients with polypharmacy and/or cognitive impairment, but it can also incur additional coordination for patient transportation and third-party coverage. On the other hand, a medication that can be safely interrupted may be a better option for patients with poor healthcare access or those with recurrent hospitalizations.

Outcome

The displaced intertrochanteric femur fracture required surgical intervention; the patient underwent cephalomedullary nail placement. Her postoperative course was complicated by blood loss anemia requiring transfusion. Due to her neurocognitive disease, she was not able to participate in physical therapy. Based on her family's wishes, she was transferred to a skilled facility with hospice benefits.

Clinical Pearls/Pitfalls
- Osteoporosis evaluation in older adults should include assessment of fall risk and frailty.
- Cognitive impairment is associated with a higher risk for falls and hip fractures.
- Polypharmacy provides an additional risk and should be addressed regularly.
- Adequate nutrition, including intake of calcium and vitamin D, is essential for musculoskeletal health in the elderly.
- A personalized exercise plan that includes muscle strengthening and resistance training can have significant musculoskeletal benefits in older adults.

References

1. Cruz-Jentoft AJ, et al. Sarcopenia: European consensus on definition and diagnosis: report of the European Working Group on Sarcopenia in Older People. Age Ageing. 2010;39(4):412–23.
2. Studenski S, et al. Gait speed and survival in older adults. JAMA. 2011;305(1):50–8.

3. Bischoff HA, et al. Identifying a cut-off point for normal mobility: a comparison of the timed "up and go" test in community-dwelling and institutionalised elderly women. Age Ageing. 2003;32(3):315–20.
4. Alley DE, et al. Grip strength cutpoints for the identification of clinically relevant weakness. J Gerontol A Biol Sci Med Sci. 2014;69(5):559–66.
5. Dodds RM, et al. Grip strength across the life course: normative data from twelve British studies. PLoS One. 2014;9(12):e113637.
6. Kiely DK, et al. Identifying nursing home residents at risk for falling. J Am Geriatr Soc. 1998;46(5):551–5.
7. Lawlor DA, Patel R, Ebrahim S. Association between falls in elderly women and chronic diseases and drug use: cross sectional study. BMJ. 2003;327(7417):712–7.
8. Ensrud KE, et al. Central nervous system-active medications and risk for falls in older women. J Am Geriatr Soc. 2002;50(10):1629–37.
9. Wu Q, et al. Selective serotonin reuptake inhibitor treatment and risk of fractures: a meta-analysis of cohort and case-control studies. Osteoporos Int. 2012;23(1):365–75.
10. Rabenda V, et al. Relationship between use of antidepressants and risk of fractures: a meta-analysis. Osteoporos Int. 2013;24(1):121–37.
11. Muir SW, Gopaul K, Montero Odasso MM. The role of cognitive impairment in fall risk among older adults: a systematic review and meta-analysis. Age Ageing. 2012;41(3):299–308.
12. Brown JS, et al. Urinary incontinence: does it increase risk for falls and fractures? Study of Osteoporotic Fractures Research Group. J Am Geriatr Soc. 2000;48(7):721–5.
13. Kanis JA, et al. FRAX and the assessment of fracture probability in men and women from the UK. Osteoporos Int. 2008;19(4):385–97.
14. Berry SD, et al. Fracture risk assessment in long-term care (FRAiL): development and validation of a prediction model. J Gerontol A Biol Sci Med Sci. 2018;73(6):763–9.
15. Visser M, Deeg DJ, Lips P. Low vitamin D and high parathyroid hormone levels as determinants of loss of muscle strength and muscle mass (sarcopenia): the Longitudinal Aging Study Amsterdam. J Clin Endocrinol Metab. 2003;88(12):5766–72.
16. Cauley JA, et al. Serum 25-hydroxyvitamin D concentrations and risk for hip fractures. Ann Intern Med. 2008;149(4):242–50.
17. Zhao JG, et al. Association between calcium or vitamin D supplementation and fracture incidence in community-dwelling older adults: a systematic review and meta-analysis. JAMA. 2017;318(24):2466–82.
18. Bischoff-Ferrari HA, et al. Effect of vitamin D on falls: a meta-analysis. JAMA. 2004;291(16):1999–2006.
19. Uusi-Rasi K, et al. Exercise and vitamin D in fall prevention among older women: a randomized clinical trial. JAMA Intern Med. 2015;175(5):703–11.

20. Reid IR. Osteoporosis: evidence for vitamin D and calcium in older people. Drug Ther Bull. 2020;58(8):122–5.
21. Guirguis-Blake JM, et al. Interventions to prevent falls in older adults: updated evidence report and systematic review for the US Preventive Services Task Force. JAMA. 2018;319(16):1705–16.
22. Sherrington C, et al. Exercise for preventing falls in older people living in the community. Cochrane Database Syst Rev. 2019;1(1):CD012424.
23. Troy KL, et al. Exercise early and often: effects of physical activity and exercise on women's bone health. Int J Environ Res Public Health. 2018;15(5):878.
24. Dent E, et al. International Clinical Practice Guidelines for Sarcopenia (ICFSR): screening, diagnosis and management. J Nutr Health Aging. 2018;22(10):1148–61.
25. WHO Guidelines Approved by the Guidelines Review Committee. Global recommendations on physical activity for health. Geneva: World Health Organization; 2010.

Relative Energy Deficiency in Sport/Functional Hypothalamic Amenorrhea

9

Katherine Haseltine and Jessica Starr

Case Presentation

A 24-year-old woman presents with secondary amenorrhea. The patient underwent menarche at age 13, with periods occurring every 1–2 months until age 18. At that time, she became vegan and increased her physical activity from 20 to 50 miles of running per week. She also began to lose weight, going from 110 pounds (BMI 22 kg/m^2) to 86 pounds (BMI 17.4 kg/m^2), and menstrual cycles stopped altogether. She did not pursue medical treatment for several years, until the age 21 when she saw a gynecologist who performed a progesterone challenge without a withdrawal bleed. She was started on oral estrogen and progesterone. She also sought counseling for disordered eating, broadened her diet, and increased her weight to 106 pounds but remained amenorrheic, prompting

K. Haseltine
Hospital for Special Surgery, New York, NY, USA
e-mail: haseltinek@hss.edu

J. Starr (✉)
Hospital for Special Surgery, New York, NY, USA

Clinical Medicine, Weill Cornell Medical College, New York, NY, USA

New York Presbyterian Hospital, New York, NY, USA
e-mail: starrj@hss.edu

current evaluation. Physical examination was notable for a thin young woman with orange discoloration of her hands, but normal dentition and no evidence of lanugo. Hormone replacement therapy was stopped, and laboratories several weeks later showed beta hCG <5, LH 4 mIU/mL (premenopausal women, follicular phase 1.9–12.5, mid-cycle peak 8.7–76.3, luteal phase 0.5–16.9 mIU/mL), FSH 4.1 mIU/mL (premenopausal women, follicular phase 2.5–10.2, mid-cycle peak 3.1–17.7, luteal phase 1.5–9.1 mIU/mL), estradiol 53 pg/mL (premenopausal women, follicular stage 39–375, mid-cycle stage 94–762, luteal stage 48–440 pg/mL), progesterone <0.5 ng/mL (premenopausal women, follicular phase <1, luteal phase 2.6–21.5 ng/mL), prolactin 5.8 ng/mL (3–30 ng/mL), TSH 1.48 mIU/L (0.40–4.50 mIU/L), and carotene 234 μg/dL (6–77 μg/dL). Repeat laboratories several months later confirmed these findings. Bone density showed Z-scores of −3.1 at the lumbar spine, −0.6 at the right femoral neck, −0.7 at the right total hip, and −1.1 at the left one-third radius.

Assessment and Diagnosis

The most likely diagnosis for a young woman presenting with secondary amenorrhea and low BMI is functional hypothalamic amenorrhea (FHA). FHA is defined as amenorrhea with low estrogen and the absence of organic abnormality. It is caused by disruption of the hypothalamic-pituitary-gonadal axis with abnormal gonadotropin-releasing hormone (GnRH) pulsatility, which in turn affects luteinizing hormone (LH) pulse amplitude, leading to low estradiol levels. FHA can result from weight loss, eating disorders, excessive exercise, or psychological stress [1].

As FHA is a diagnosis of exclusion, it is important to rule out other causes of secondary amenorrhea. Basic evaluation begins with a serum pregnancy test. Clinicians should also perform a careful review of medications for recent oral contraceptive use or psychiatric medications that could cause hyperprolactinemia. Physical examination should focus on evaluation for possible eating disorders, which may present with bradycardia, hypothermia, loss of dental enamel, salivary gland enlargement, cool extremities, lanugo (fine body hair), and hypercarotenemia. Other differential diagnoses that should be ruled out by thorough history, physical examination, and laboratories include sellar mass, polycystic ovarian syndrome, premature ovarian insufficiency, and intrauterine adhesions.

In this patient presented in the preceding vignette, history revealed restrictive eating behavior in the setting of high levels of physical activity. Together with her history of low bone mineral density, her presentation is most consistent with a type of FHA called relative energy deficiency in sport (RED-S). RED-S is adapted from the Female Athlete Triad, which includes women with irregular periods, low energy availability, and low BMD. RED-S is a syndrome affecting multiple layers of physiologic function that can affect both male and female athletes. It is caused by an imbalance between dietary intake and energy expenditure, leading to inadequate energy for maintenance of health and optimal functioning [2–4].

In addition to hypogonadism, patients with RED-S often have additional hormonal alterations including higher cortisol levels, higher ghrelin (orexigenic), lower leptin (anorexigenic), and lower insulin-like growth factor 1 (IGF-1) than their peers (Fig. 9.1) [5, 6].

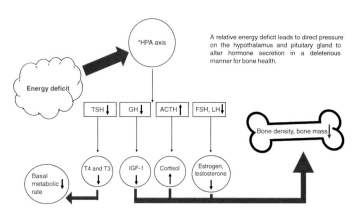

Fig. 9.1 Key endocrine hormones in RED-S. *HPA = hypothalamic-pituitary adrenal

Low BMD is a primary concern in FHA and in RED-S in particular. Patients with onset of FHA during adolescent years may fail to attain peak bone mass, which can be compounded by ongoing bone loss. Studies comparing bone density in eumenorrheic and amenorrheic athletes have demonstrated significantly lower BMD in women with menstrual disturbances, as well as an increased risk of stress fractures. The etiology is multifactorial, stemming from hypoestrogenism, nutritional deficiencies, elevated cortisol levels, and low IGF-1. Low testosterone may also contribute to bone loss in both females and males [7–10].

Identification of RED-S in men is less common than in women, although men participating in endurance sports with high energy expenditure or in weight-sensitive sports such as wrestling, boxing, and rowing are at risk. A lower rate of diagnosis may be due to the fact that hypogonadism can be more difficult to recognize in men and that many clinicians are unfamiliar with the diagnosis. Further research in this area is needed [10].

Management

FHA is often challenging to treat and requires an interdisciplinary approach between nutritionists, mental health providers, and the medical team. The primary objective is to correct the energy imbalance by encouraging increased caloric intake and moderating exercise. It is common for patients to be resistant to therapy: it often requires weight gain, and for RED-S patients, it can require drastically reducing or ceasing athletic endeavors. In patients with severe electrolyte abnormalities, bradycardia, or hypotension, inpatient treatment may be necessary [5].

For those with a mild presentation, nutritional counseling can be sufficient. Cognitive behavioral therapy (CBT) is another non-pharmacologic intervention that has proven effective for FHA—women treated with CBT are more likely to recover ovarian activity and have been noted to have lower cortisol, higher leptin, and higher TSH than those treated with observation alone [11].

In terms of pharmacologic therapy, clinicians should start by ensuring that patients are receiving adequate amounts of calcium and vitamin D. Current recommendations state that optimal calcium intake for amenorrheic athletes is 1500 mg/day, as opposed to 1200 mg/day for healthy, menstruating teenagers and young adults [12]. Ideally, most of the 1500 mg/day of calcium should come from food sources rather than supplements, which have variable absorption. Children and young adults require at least 600 IU/day of vitamin D, and titration based on serum 25-hydroxyvitamin D levels is often necessary [13]. Vitamin D is less readily available from food than calcium and should be taken in supplement form if the patient is found to be deficient.

Treatment with oral contraceptive pills (OCPs) for resumption of menses or low BMD is not recommended, as there are no strong data for a protective effect on bone, perhaps due to the downregulation of the bone-trophic hormone, IGF-1, by ethinyl estradiol-containing OCPs. For women who have ongoing amenorrhea despite a reasonable trial of conservative measures (approximately 6–12 months), short-term treatment with transdermal estradiol and cyclic progesterone is appropriate [5, 14].

The use of bisphosphonates in patients with low BMD is not recommended. There is not strong evidence for efficacy, and significant concern exists for teratogenicity in women of reproductive age. Similar concerns are present for denosumab, which has not been studied in premenopausal women and may also pose a risk for teratogenicity. In rare, severe cases such as patients with very low BMD and delayed fracture healing, recombinant parathyroid hormone can be considered, although failure to correct the underlying energy deficit will likely blunt the efficacy of PTH therapy [5].

Outcome

With weight gain and reduction in exercise, the patient resumed menses after several months. She remains off hormone replacement therapy and continues to work closely with a nutritionist and mental health provider. Repeat bone density showed modest improvement.

Clinical Pearls/Pitfalls
- Functional hypothalamic amenorrhea (FHA) is secondary amenorrhea due to low energy availability or stress and is a diagnosis of exclusion.
- Relative energy deficiency in sport (RED-S) is a type of FHA present in athletes with a variety of physiologic impairments including low BMD.
- FHA can be difficult to treat and often requires a multidisciplinary team.
- Oral contraceptive pills, bisphosphonates, and denosumab should not routinely be used as treatments for FHA, but rather the focus of therapy should remain to correct the energy deficit.

References

1. Caronia LM, Martin C, Welt CK, Sykiotis GP, Quinton R, Thambundit A, Avbelj M, Dhruvakumar S, Plummer L, Hughes VA, Seminara SB, Boepple PA, Sidis Y, Crowley WF Jr, Martin KA, Hall JE, Pitteloud N. A genetic basis for functional hypothalamic amenorrhea. N Engl J Med. 2011;364(3):215–25.
2. Mountjoy M, Sundgot-Borgen J, Burke L, et al. The IOC consensus statement: beyond the Female Athlete Triad—Relative Energy Deficiency in Sport (RED-S). Br J Sports Med. 2014;48:491–7.
3. Mountjoy M, Sundgot-Borgen JK, Burke LM, et al. IOC consensus statement on relative energy deficiency in sport (RED-S): 2018 update. Br J Sports Med. 2018;52:687–97.
4. De Souza MJ, Williams NI, Nattiv A, et al. Misunderstanding the female athlete triad: refuting the IOC consensus statement on Relative Energy Deficiency in Sport (RED-S). Br J Sports Med. 2014;48:1461–5.
5. Gordon CM, Ackerman KE, Berga SL, Kaplan JR, Mastorakos G, Misra M, Murad MH, Santoro NF, Warren MP. Functional hypothalamic amenorrhea: an Endocrine Society clinical practice guideline. J Clin Endocrinol Metab. 2017;102(5):1413–39. https://doi.org/10.1210/jc.2017-00131.
6. Logue D, Madigan SM, Delahunt E, et al. Low energy availability in athletes: a review of prevalence, dietary patterns, physiological health, and sports performance. Sports Med. 2018;48:73–96. https://doi-org.ezproxy.med.cornell.edu/10.1007/s40279-017-0790-3.

7. Warren MP, Perlroth NE. The effects of intense exercise on the female reproductive system. J Endocrinol. 2001;170(1):3–11. https://doi.org/10.1677/joe.0.1700003. PMID: 11431132.
8. Barrack MT, Gibbs JC, De Souza MJ, Williams NI, Nichols JF, Rauh MJ, Nattiv A. Higher incidence of bone stress injuries with increasing female athlete triad-related risk factors: a prospective multisite study of exercising girls and women. Am J Sports Med. 2014;42(4):949–58. https://doi.org/10.1177/0363546513520295. Epub 2014 Feb 24. PMID: 24567250.
9. Christo K, Prabhakaran R, Lamparello B, et al. Bone metabolism in adolescent athletes with amenorrhea, athletes with eumenorrhea, and control subjects. Pediatrics. 2008;121(6):1127–36. https://doi.org/10.1542/peds.2007-2392.
10. Tenforde AS, Barrack MT, Nattiv A, Fredericson M. Parallels with the female athlete triad in male athletes. Sports Med. 2016;46(2):171–82. https://doi.org/10.1007/s40279-015-0411-y. PMID: 26497148.
11. Michopoulos V, Mancini F, Loucks TL, Berga SL. Neuroendocrine recovery initiated by cognitive behavioral therapy in women with functional hypothalamic amenorrhea: a randomized, controlled trial. Fertil Steril. 2013;99(7):2084–91.e1. https://doi.org/10.1016/j.fertnstert.2013.02.036.
12. Kunstel K. Calcium requirements for the athlete. Curr Sports Med Rep. 2005;4(4):203–6. https://doi.org/10.1097/01.CSMR.0000306208.56939.01.
13. Holick MF, Binkley NC, Bischoff-Ferrari HA, Gordon CM, Hanley DA, Heaney RP, Murad MH, Weaver CM. Evaluation, treatment, and prevention of vitamin D deficiency: an Endocrine Society clinical practice guideline. J Clin Endocrinol Metab. 2011;96(7):1911–30.
14. Altayar O, Al Nofal A, Carranza Leon BG, Prokop LJ, Wang Z, Murad MH. Treatments to prevent bone loss in functional hypothalamic amenorrhea: a systematic review and meta-analysis. J Endocr Soc. 2017;1(5):500–11. Published 2017 Apr 26. https://doi.org/10.1210/js.2017-00102.

Chronic Kidney Disease – Mineral and Bone Disorder (CKD-MBD)

10

Valerie S. Barta, Maria V. DeVita, and Jordan L. Rosenstock

Case Presentation

A 62-year-old woman with chronic kidney disease stage 4 (CKD 4) due to uncontrolled hypertension and diabetes mellitus type 2 is referred for evaluation of elevated parathyroid hormone (PTH). She has had mild diffuse skin itching over the last few months but otherwise feels well without history of bone pain or fractures. On physical exam, she has full range of motion and strength in her joints and extremities. There is no joint inflammation or bony abnormalities. Her skin is well perfused and without rash. Her laboratories are pertinent for serum creatinine 3.2 mg/dL, estimated glomerular filtration rate (eGFR) 20 mL/min, bicarbonate ($HCO_3)^-$ 19 mmol/L (22–31 mmol/L), phosphate 6.2 mg/dL (2.5–4.5 mg/dL), 25-hydroxyvitamin D 18 ng/mL (30–80 ng/mL), 1,25-dihydroxyvitamin D (calcitriol or [1,25-$(OH)_2$-D]) 20 pg/mL (19.9–79.3 pg/mL), calcium (Ca^{2+}) 8.2 mg/dL (8.4–10.5 mg/

V. S. Barta (✉) · M. V. DeVita · J. L. Rosenstock
Division of Nephrology, Lenox Hill Hospital, Donald and Barbara Zucker School of Medicine at Hofstra/Northwell, New York, NY, USA
e-mail: vbarta@northwell.edu; mdevita@northwell.edu; jrosenstock@northwell.edu

© The Author(s), under exclusive license to Springer Nature Switzerland AG 2021
N. E. Cusano (ed.), *Osteoporosis*,
https://doi.org/10.1007/978-3-030-83951-2_10

dL), albumin 4.0 g/dL, intact PTH 375 pg/mL (15–65 pg/mL), and bone-specific alkaline phosphatase (BALP) 75 µg/L (4–36 µg/L). A CT scan performed 2 months previously showed coronary artery calcifications.

Assessment and Diagnosis

Chronic kidney disease with mineral and bone disorder (CKD-MBD) describes the systemic alterations in mineral, metabolic, hormonal, and bone homeostasis that can increase the risk of fractures, vascular calcification, cardiovascular morbidity, and mortality in patients with eGFR <60 mL/min. Patients with CKD are 2–17 times more likely to experience bone fracture than the general population. This risk increases proportionately as kidney function declines, with most CKD patients stages three to five showing signs of high bone turnover and increased PTH [1, 2]. Rates of hip fracture in end-stage kidney disease (ESKD) have increased over the last 30 years. CKD patients with bone fractures have decreased quality of life, longer hospitalizations, incur higher healthcare costs, and experience a 16–60% increase in morbidity and mortality compared to patients who fracture with normal kidney function [3]. CKD-MBD affects bone and mineral metabolism in three main areas: serum mineral and hormone imbalance, decreased bone quality and strength, and increased extraskeletal calcifications.

Serum biomarkers used to assess CKD-MBD include phosphate, 1,25-dihydroxyvitamin D, calcium, bicarbonate, PTH, and fibroblast growth factor-23 (FGF-23) (Table 10.1). As eGFR declines, phosphate clearance is reduced, triggering the rise in phosphaturic hormones PTH and FGF-23 in a feedback loop to increase kidney excretion of phosphate. Hyperphosphatemia and elevated FGF-23 along with reduced kidney function result in low 1,25-dihydroxyvitamin D which causes hypocalcemia, yet another trigger for PTH release. Chronic overproduction of parathyroid hormone results in the typical high turnover bone disease seen in these patients (Fig. 10.1). Additionally, metabolic acidosis is frequent in CKD and directly causes bone loss, impaired bone mineralization, and increased FGF-23 (Table 10.1) [4].

Table 10.1 Serum biomarkers of CKD-MBD

	↑ [Phosphate]	↓ [1,25-(OH)$_2$-D]	↓ [Calcium]	↑ [FGF-23]	↑ [PTH]	↓ [HCO3-]
Driven by	CKD (reduced ability of the kidney to excrete Phosphate)	↑ FGF-23 ↑ Phosphate ↓ Calcidiol conversion to calcitriol due to CKD and FGF-23 (via ↓ renal tubular 1α hydroxylase)	↓ 1,25-(OH)$_2$D	↑ Phosphate ↑ PTH Metabolic acidosis	↑ Phosphate ↓ 1,25-(OH)$_2$D ↓ Ca^{2+}	CKD (reduced ability of the kidney to generate ammonia and excrete H+)
Results in	↑ PTH ↑ FGF23 ↓ 1,25-(OH)$_2$-D ↑ CVD + mortality	↓ Ca^{2+} ↑ PTH	↑ PTH	↑ Kidney phosphate excretion ↓ Renal tubular 1α hydroxylase Parathyroid hyperplasia ↓ Bone formation and mineralization ↓ BALP ↑ CVD + mortality	↑ Kidney phosphate excretion ↑ FGF-23 Parathyroid hyperplasia ↑ Bone resorption ↑ Bone formation ↑ CVD + mortality	↑ FGF23 ↓ Bone formation ↑ Bone resorption

CVD = cardiovascular disease

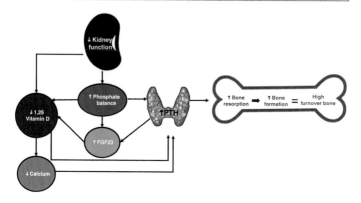

Fig. 10.1 Drivers of secondary hyperparathyroidism in CKD-MBD

Renal osteodystrophy is a broad term describing the various effects of CKD-MBD on bone formation and resorption. Bone morphology in CKD is mainly impacted by the rate of bone turnover; degree of bone mineralization and bone volume play a lesser role. The net effect of the abovementioned mineral/hormone imbalance is a PTH-induced increase in bone resorption (coupled with increased bone formation) leading to higher rates of bone turnover. The type and degree of renal osteodystrophy depend on the combination of these factors and the guideline-derived medical interventions initiated in response to abnormal serum biomarkers (Fig. 10.2). In early CKD, bone turnover rates tend to be high, driven by secondary hyperparathyroidism. As CKD progresses to ESKD, low bone turnover is more prevalent [1]. This may partially be iatrogenic, due to over-suppression of PTH by medications such as calcium-based phosphate binders, activated vitamin D, and calcimimetics.

The third component of CKD-MBD is extraskeletal calcification. Accelerated vascular calcification is one of the strongest predictors of cardiovascular events and mortality in CKD [5]. Hyperphosphatemia has been consistently shown to increase mortality, likely due to its direct calcifying effect on coronary vessels and valves [6]. Many other mineral and hormonal altera-

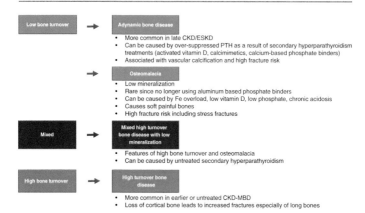

Fig. 10.2 Four types of renal osteodystrophy

tions in CKD-MBD and their treatments have been associated with increased vascular calcification, cardiovascular events, and mortality, including hypercalcemia, the use of calcium-based phosphate binders, high FGF-23, and both high and low PTH [7–9]. Calcimimetics such as cinacalcet that reduce PTH and calcium levels may possibly reduce vascular calcification risk in ESKD [10]. Calciphylaxis is a rare but often deadly condition associated with CKD-MBD seen almost exclusively in advanced CKD/ESKD. It is thought to be caused by hydroxyapatite deposition within vessel layers and surrounding subcutaneous adipose tissue resulting in painful skin ulcerations that turn necrotic and are easily infected. These patients need immediate referral to a multidisciplinary care team including a nephrologist, vascular surgeon, and dermatologist, as the 1-year mortality rate is greater than 50% [11].

Management

The management of CKD-MBD is centered on preventing the adverse consequences associated with secondary hyperparathyroidism.

Hyperphosphatemia

- Low phosphate diet
- Phosphate binders

Hyperphosphatemia drives secondary hyperparathyroidism, increased serum FGF-23, and inhibits vitamin D activation in CKD. As such, an important early intervention in CKD-MBD is counseling the patient on dietary phosphate restriction, less than 800–1000 mg/day, to keep phosphate "toward normal range" [12]. Controlling phosphate intake can be challenging for patients. The typical American diet includes highly processed foods with large amounts of inorganic phosphate additives. These foods contain nearly 60% more phosphate than similar organic sources without additives, and inorganic phosphate is 100% bioavailable [13]. Two recent trials have shown that dietary guidance on removing foods containing phosphate additives in ESKD patients led to significantly lower serum phosphate levels [14, 15]. Plant-based sources of dietary phosphate, such as grains and legumes, are less bioavailable than natural animal-based sources like dairy, and both of these natural phosphate sources are less bioavailable than foods with inorganic phosphate additives [16, 17].

While dietary control is imperative in hyperphosphatemia, inorganic phosphate additives are ubiquitous and difficult to avoid. Patients will often need medication to help reduce their serum phosphate. Calcium-containing phosphate binders (calcium carbonate and calcium acetate) are the most frequently used worldwide as they are readily available and affordable. However, guidelines now suggest "restricting the dose" of calcium-based binders due to their association with adynamic bone disease, vascular calcification, and mortality, likely attributable to the calcium component [12, 16]. Non-calcium-based binders (sevelamer carbonate and sevelamer hydrochloride) are the most common alternatives; however, like calcium-based binders, their use is limited by pill burden, compliance, and gastrointestinal side effects. Newer phosphate binders contain iron (sucroferric oxyhydroxide and ferric citrate) which have the additional benefit of improving anemia which is common in CKD patients. A recent trial showed that sucroferric oxyhydroxide slowed vascular calcification in dialysis patients [18]. Intestinal phosphate transport inhibitors, tenapanor and nicotinamide, are currently in preclinical testing. Rather than binding gut phosphorous each meal, these agents block paracellular transport of phosphate, reducing intestinal absorption [17]. How these agents will compare to phosphate binders in terms of efficacy, gastrointestinal side effects, and decreased pill burden remains to be determined.

Secondary Hyperparathyroidism

- Decrease serum phosphate
- Increase 25-hydroxyvitamin D and 1,25-dihydroxyvitamin D
- Decrease PTH with activated vitamin D and/or calcimimetics

The optimal PTH level in CKD is not known. KDIGO suggests reducing "progressively rising or persistently elevated" PTH [12]. Lowering PTH in secondary hyperparathyroidism involves normalizing serum phosphate and repleting both nutritional 25-hydroxyvitamin D deficiency and acquired 1,25-dihydroxyvitamin D deficiency. Activated vitamin D (calcitriol or its analogs doxercalciferol, paricalcitol, and alfacalcidol) is frequently used to effectively lower PTH. These medications can result in hypercalcemia, increased intestinal phosphate absorption, and over-suppression of PTH, so careful attention to dosing and monitoring of serum calcium, phosphate, and PTH levels is prudent [19, 20]. Current guidelines suggest using activated vitamin D only in patients with CKD 4, 5, and ESKD who have "severe and progressive hyperparathyroidism" [12].

Calcimimetics such as cinacalcet or etelcalcetide can be used as an alternative to or in conjunction with activated vitamin D to treat secondary hyperparathyroidism, but they are currently only approved for use in ESKD. Calcimimetics suppress PTH secretion by binding the calcium-sensing receptor on the parathyroid gland. They effectively control PTH in dialysis patients and are especially useful in patients who have hypercalcemia and hyperphosphatemia which limit the use of activated vitamin D. However, despite cinacalcet effectively lowering PTH in a large trial of dialysis patients with severe hyperparathyroidism, there was no reduction in fracture risk or cardiovascular events [21]. Multiple gland parathyroidectomy is ultimately recommended for those with severe hyperparathyroidism who do not respond to or who develop contraindications to medical therapy [12].

Chronic Metabolic Acidosis

Metabolic acidosis is extremely common among CKD patients and can directly contribute to bone loss. Acutely, the bone buffers acid, releasing calcium. Chronic metabolic acidosis tilts the bone turnover scale toward increased resorption and decreased bone formation. It also increases osteoblast production of FGF-23 which further decreases bone formation as well as mineralization [4]. There have been accumulating data that treating metabolic acidosis may slow the progression of kidney disease [22], so CKD guidelines recommend administering base when the serum bicarbonate is less than 22 meq/L. [23] Whether treating metabolic acidosis in CKD improves bone disease has not yet been specifically studied. We treat metabolic acidosis in CKD with a reduced acid diet (lower animal protein) and oral sodium bicarbonate. A new agent, veverimer, that acts as a hydrogen and chloride binder in the gastrointestinal tract, is under investigation for treating metabolic acidosis in CKD and has shown efficacy in early studies [24], although bone effects have not been evaluated.

Osteoporosis

- Assess bone mineral density in CKD 3–5 and ESRD with DXA
- Assess bone turnover, using PTH and bone-specific alkaline phosphatase

- If high bone turnover, consider these agents:
  - Bisphosphonates (dose caution, nephrotoxicity of intravenous forms)
  - Denosumab (monitoring for hypocalcemia)
- If low bone turnover, consider osteoanabolic agents

It is suggested that any CKD patient with evidence of renal osteodystrophy and fracture should be considered as having osteoporosis, as their bone quality and strength are similarly impaired [1]. New to KDIGO guidelines in 2017, the use of DXA to determine BMD is now recommended in patients with CKD 3 and up, who have "evidence of CKD-MBD or risk factors for osteoporosis" [12]. Treating low BMD in CKD first involves assessing the degree of bone turnover. While a bone biopsy is the gold standard in assessing bone turnover and quality, it is an invasive and lengthy process that is rarely performed clinically [25, 26]. Measuring bone turnover markers such as PTH and BALP is a more practical way to assess bone turnover rates, though these have limitations [1, 27, 28]. Significantly high PTH and BALP levels in CKD patients correlate with high bone turnover, and significantly low levels correlate to low bone turnover states. Unfortunately, intermediate levels are difficult to interpret, and a bone biopsy would be ideal in such patients [1].

Treatment of osteoporosis in CKD can be challenging. Bisphosphonates are cleared by the kidney resulting in a prolonged blood half-life, although this is dwarfed by the bone half-life so the clinical implications are unclear [29]. Nephrotoxicity has been reported, particularly with intravenous agents. Pamidronate is associated with focal glomerular sclerosis (especially with multiple high doses), and zoledronic acid has been reported to cause acute tubular injury even at the 4 mg dose [29, 30]. However, recent data suggest that with careful attention to dosing, infusion rates, and treatment frequency in CKD, nephrotoxicity is rare [1]. Denosumab is not cleared by the kidney; however, serum calcium needs to be monitored frequently posttreatment as it can cause severe hypocalcemia in CKD [31]. While bisphosphonates should be avoided in low bone turnover disease, osteoanabolic agents are likely useful in this setting [1]. Teriparatide has been studied in small numbers of patients with

ESKD and low bone turnover [32, 33]. Abaloparatide may have an advantage over teriparatide in that it is less likely to cause hypercalcemia, but this has not been tested in CKD [34].

Outcome

We educated our patient to avoid highly bioavailable dietary phosphate loads, such as processed foods with inorganic phosphate additives (e.g., canned food, dark sodas/colas, deli meat), as well as animal-derived phosphate sources including dairy. At her follow-up visit, her serum phosphate remained above normal, and she admitted to struggling with limiting her milk consumption. Sevelamer carbonate was initiated at 800 mg three times daily with meals to bind dietary phosphate in the gut and limit its absorption, with the goal of returning serum phosphate toward normal levels.

We started cholecalciferol 5000 IU daily, achieving a 25-hydroxyvitamin D level of 40 ng/mL. On follow-up, her 1,25-dihydroxyvitamin D and calcium levels remained in the low normal range; however, her PTH was still quite elevated at 288 pg/mL. Calcitriol 0.25 μg 3× weekly was started, which increased her 1,25-dihydroxyvitamin D and calcium levels to the mid-normal range, and reduced PTH to 109 pg/mL.

We added sodium bicarbonate tablets of 650 mg three times daily to our patient's regimen, with improvement in serum HCO_3- level to 23 mEq/L.

Clinical Pearls/Pitfalls
- Most patients with chronic kidney disease (CKD) 3 through end-stage kidney disease have some degree of chronic kidney disease-mineral and bone disorder (CKD-MBD).
- Preventing or delaying progressive metabolic and bone complications is essential to reducing the high morbidity and mortality rates associated with CKD-MBD.
- In patients with CKD, careful monitoring of bone and mineral abnormalities can represent opportunities to reduce risk of fractures, cardiovascular events, and mortality.

References

1. Damasiewicz MJ, Nickolas TL. Rethinking bone disease in kidney disease. JBMR Plus. 2018;2(6):309–22.
2. Pimentel A, Ureña-Torres P, Zillikens MC, Bover J, Cohen-Solal M. Fractures in patients with CKD—diagnosis, treatment, and prevention: a review by members of the European Calcified Tissue Society and the European Renal Association of Nephrology Dialysis and Transplantation. Kidney Int. 2017;92:1343–55.
3. Floege J, Drüeke TB. Mineral and bone disorder in chronic kidney disease: pioneering studies. Kidney Int. 2020;98:807–11.
4. Bushinsky DA. Acidosis and renal bone disease. In: Olgaard K, Salusk IB, Silver J, editors. *The spectrum of mineral and bone disorders in chronic kidney disease*. 2nd ed. Oxford University Press; 2010. p. 253–65.
5. Liu M, Li XC, Lu L, et al. Cardiovascular disease and its relationship with chronic kidney disease. Eur Rev Med Pharmacol Sci. 2014;19:2918–26.
6. Block GA, Raggi P, Bellasi A, Kooienga L, Spiegel DM. Mortality effect of coronary calcification and phosphate binder choice in incident hemodialysis patients. Kidney Int. 2007;71(5):438–41.
7. Palmer SC, Hayen A, Macaskill P, et al. Serum levels of phosphorus, parathyroid hormone, and calcium and risks of death and cardiovascular disease in individuals with chronic kidney disease a systematic review and meta-analysis. JAMA. 2011;305(11):1119–27.
8. Hu MC, Shi M, Zhang J, et al. Klotho deficiency causes vascular calcification in chronic kidney disease. J Am Soc Nephrol. 2011;22(1):124–36.
9. Shantouf R, Kovesdy CP, Kim Y, et al. Association of serum alkaline phosphatase with coronary artery calcification in maintenance hemodialysis patients. Clin J Am Soc Nephrol. 2009;4(6):1106–14.
10. Ureña-Torres PA, Floege J, Hawley CM, et al. Protocol adherence and the progression of cardiovascular calcification in the ADVANCE study. Nephrol Dial Transplant. 2013;28(1):146–52.
11. Nigwekar SU, Zhao S, Wenger J, et al. A nationally representative study of calcific uremic arteriolopathy risk factors. J Am Soc Nephrol. 2016;27(11):3421–9.
12. Kidney Disease: Improving Global Outcomes (KDIGO) CKD-MBD Update Work Group. KDIGO 2017 clinical practice guideline update for the diagnosis, evaluation, prevention and treatment of chronic kidney disease-mineral and bone disorder CKD-MBD. Kidney Int Suppl. 2017;7(1):1–59. https://kdigo.org/wp-content/uploads/2017/02/2017-KDIGO-CKD-MBD-GL-Update.pdf. Published 2017. Accessed March 20, 2021.
13. Cooke A. Dietary food-additive phosphate and human health outcomes. Compr Rev Food Sci Food Saf. 2014;16(5):906–1021.

14. Sullivan C, Sayre SS, Leon JB, et al. Effect of food additives on hyper-phosphatemia among patients with end-stage renal disease: a randomized controlled trial. JAMA. 2009;301(6):629–35.

15. de Fornasari MLL, dos Santos Sens YA. Replacing phosphorus-containing food additives with foods without additives reduces phosphatemia in end-stage renal disease patients: a randomized clinical trial. J Ren Nutr. 2017;27(2):97–105.

16. Barreto FC, Barreto DV, Massy ZA, Drüeke TB. Strategies for phosphate control in patients with CKD. Kidney Int Rep. 2019;4(8):1043–56.

17. Cozzolino M, Ketteler M, Wagner CA. An expert update on novel thera-peutic targets for hyperphosphatemia in chronic kidney disease: preclini-cal and clinical innovations. Expert Opin Ther Targets. 2020;24(5):477–88. https://doi.org/10.1080/14728222.2020.1743680.

18. Isaka Y, Hamano T, Fujii H, et al. Optimal phosphate control related to coronary artery calcification in dialysis patients. J Am Soc Nephrol. 2021;32(3):723–35.

19. Wang AYM, Fang F, Chan J, et al. Effect of paricalcitol on left ventricular mass and function in CKD-the OPERA trial. J Am Soc Nephrol. 2014;25:175–86.

20. Thadhani R, Appelbaum E, Pritchett Y, et al. Vitamin D therapy and car-diac structure and function in patients with chronic kidney disease: the PRIMO randomized controlled trial. JAMA. 2012;307(7):674–84.

21. EVOLVE Trial Investigators, Chertow GM, Block GA, Correa-Rotter R, et al. Effect of cinacalcet on cardiovascular disease in patients undergoing dialysis. N Engl J Med. 2012;367:2482–94.

22. Navaneethan SD, Shao J, Buysse J, Bushinsky D. Effects of treatment of metabolic acidosis in CKD a systematic review and meta-analysis. Clin J Am Soc Nephrol. 2019;14(7):1011–20.

23. Andrassy KM. KDIGO 2012 clinical practice guideline for the evaluation and management of chronic kidney disease. Kidney Int. 2013;3(1):1–116.

24. Adrogué HJ, Madias NE. Veverimer: an emerging potential treatment option for managing the metabolic acidosis of CKD. Am J Kidney Dis. 2020;76(6):861–7.

25. Evenepoel P, Cunningham J, Ferrari S, et al. European Consensus Statement on the diagnosis and management of osteoporosis in chronic kidney disease stages G4-G5D. Nephrol Dial Transplant. 2021;36:42–59.

26. Nickolas TL. The quest for better biomarkers of bone turnover in CKD. J Am Soc Nephrol. 2018;29:1353–5.

27. Sprague SM, Bellorin-Font E, Jorgetti V, et al. Diagnostic accuracy of bone turnover markers and bone histology in patients with CKD treated by dialysis. Am J Kidney Dis. 2016;67(4):559–66.

28. Salam S, Gallagher O, Gossiel F, Paggiosi M, Khwaja A, Eastell R. Diagnostic accuracy of biomarkers and imaging for bone turnover in renal osteodystrophy. J Am Soc Nephrol. 2018;29(5):1557–65.

29. Damasiewicz MJ, Nickolas TL. Bisphosphonate therapy in CKD: the current state of affairs. Curr Opin Nephrol Hypertens. 2020;29(2):221–6.
30. Markowitz GS, Fine PL, Stack JI, et al. Toxic acute tubular necrosis following treatment with zoledronate (Zometa). Kidney Int. 2003;64(1):281–9.
31. Dave V, Chiang CY, Booth J, Mount PF. Hypocalcemia post denosumab in patients with chronic kidney disease stage 4-5. Am J Nephrol. 2015;41(2):129–37.
32. Cejka D, Kodras K, Bader T, Haas M. Treatment of hemodialysis-associated adynamic bone disease with teriparatide (PTH1-34): a pilot study. Kidney Blood Press Res. 2010;33:221–6.
33. Sumida K, Ubara Y, Hoshino J, et al. Once-weekly teriparatide in hemodialysis patients with hypoparathyroidism and low bone mass: a prospective study. Osteoporos Int. 2016;27(4):1441–50.
34. Miller P, et al. Effect of abaloparatide vs placebo on new vertebral fractures in postmenopausal women with osteoporosis: a randomized clinical trial. JAMA. 2017;316(7):722–33.

Antiresorptive Therapy for Osteoporosis

11

Swetha Murthi and Emilia Pauline Liao

Case Presentation

A 68-year-old postmenopausal woman with history of seizure disorder currently on carbamazepine presented to endocrine clinic for evaluation of osteoporosis. She sustained a traumatic left wrist fracture 12 years ago, with no history of falls or other fragility fractures in recent years. She had a height loss of 2 inches of unknown duration. She had no history of kidney stones, thyroid, or parathyroid disease. She had lactose intolerance which limited her dietary calcium intake. There was no family history of bone disease or fracture. Physical examination was unremarkable. Laboratories were significant for 25-hydroxyvitamin D 11.5 ng/mL, alkaline phosphatase 127 U/L (normal, 40–120 U/L), and serum cross-linked N-terminal telopeptide 24.1 (normal, 6.2–19 nmol BCE/mmol Cr). Calcium, PTH, TSH, eGFR, and 1,25-dihydroxyvitamin D levels were within normal limits. DXA showed T-scores of −2.9 at the lumbar spine, −2.0 at the left femoral neck, −2.7 at the right femoral neck, and −3.3 at the distal radius. She was started on calcium and vitamin D supplementation. What are the pharmacologic treatment options for this patient?

S. Murthi · E. P. Liao (✉)
Northwell Health Lenox Hill Hospital, New York, NY, USA
e-mail: eliao@northwell.edu

© The Author(s), under exclusive license to Springer Nature Switzerland AG 2021
N. E. Cusano (ed.), *Osteoporosis*,
https://doi.org/10.1007/978-3-030-83951-2_11

Management

Osteoporosis treatment includes both nonpharmacologic and pharmacologic therapy. Nonpharmacologic treatment includes adequate calcium and vitamin D intake, cessation of smoking, limitation of alcohol intake, fall prevention techniques, and weight-bearing exercises [1].

Pharmacologic treatment options fall into two categories: antiresorptive agents (those that mainly act to decrease bone resorption) and osteoanabolic agents (those that mainly act to increase bone formation). Antiresorptive agents include bisphosphonates, denosumab, estrogen/hormone replacement therapy, and selective estrogen receptor modulators [2]. Osteoanabolic agents include PTH and PTHrP analogs, teriparatide and abaloparatide (Chap. 13). Romosozumab is a monoclonal antibody against sclerostin that both increases bone formation and decreases bone resorption (Chap. 14). In this chapter, we will review antiresorptive agents in further detail.

Bisphosphonates (BPs)

Bisphosphonates (BPs) are antiresorptive agents that inhibit osteoclastic bone resorption by binding to hydroxyapatite-binding sites on bony surfaces that are undergoing active resorption. They also reduce osteoclast progenitor cell development and recruitment and promote osteoclast apoptosis, thereby reducing osteoclast activity.

The bisphosphonate class includes alendronate, ibandronate, risedronate, and zoledronic acid. Pamidronate, etidronate, and clodronate are no longer commonly used. Alendronate, risedronate, and ibandronate are available as oral medications for daily or weekly dosing (alendronate and risedronate) or monthly dosing (risedronate and ibandronate). Intravenous (IV) formulations include ibandronate every 3 months and zoledronic acid for annual infusion [3].

Alendronate, risedronate, and zoledronic acid improve bone mineral density and reduce vertebral and nonvertebral fracture risk. Although ibandronate was shown to reduce vertebral fractures, there was no effect on nonvertebral fracture risk in the pivotal clinical trial [1]. The American Association of Clinical Endocrinology and Endocrine Society guidelines recommend BPs, excluding ibandronate, as a first-line treatment option for osteoporosis in postmenopausal women and men and for glucocorticoid-induced osteoporosis [4, 5].

Alendronate is FDA approved for treatment of postmenopausal osteoporosis, male osteoporosis, and glucocorticoid-induced osteoporosis. The pivotal Fracture Intervention Trial (FIT) demonstrated a significant reduction in the incidence of vertebral fractures with alendronate therapy for 3–4 years [6]. There were reductions in radiographic vertebral (RR 0.52, 95% CI 0.42–0.66), clinical vertebral (RR 0.55, 95% CI 0.36–0.82), hip (RR 0.47, 95% CI 0.26–0.79), and all clinical fractures (RR 0.70, 95% CI 0.59–0.82), with significant reductions in clinical fracture risk noted by 12 months into the trial. In a meta-analysis of 11 trials of alendronate versus placebo, alendronate demonstrated reductions in vertebral fractures in patients both with and without a previous history of fracture (RR 0.55 for both), in addition to hip (RR 0.47) and nonvertebral (RR 0.77) fractures [7].

Similar to alendronate, risedronate has also been FDA approved for postmenopausal osteoporosis, male osteoporosis, and glucocorticoid-induced osteoporosis and has demonstrated efficacy for vertebral, hip, and nonvertebral fractures. In a meta-analysis of eight randomized trials of risedronate versus placebo, risedronate reduced the risk of vertebral (RR 0.64) and nonvertebral (RR 0.73) fractures [8]. In the Fosamax Actonel Comparison Trial international study (FACTS) with 12-month extension, a randomized control trial of alendronate versus risedronate, alendronate had greater BMD gains and reduction in bone turnover markers when compared to risedronate, with no significant change in upper gastrointestinal tolerability [9]. Fracture outcomes were not measured.

Zoledronic acid, a third-generation bisphosphonate, is approved for use in postmenopausal osteoporosis, male osteoporosis, and glucocorticoid-induced osteoporosis. The Health Outcomes and Reduced Incidence with Zoledronic Acid Once Yearly (HORIZON) Pivotal Fracture Trial compared zoledronic acid to placebo over a 3-year period and demonstrated a decrease in morphometric vertebral fractures by 70%, hip fractures by 41%, and nonvertebral fractures by 25% [10]. As an annual infusion, it is a convenient and effective treatment option that may have an advantage over other agents for patients for whom treatment adherence or gastrointestinal intolerance may be an issue [11].

Contraindications for BPs include known hypersensitivity, esophageal abnormalities, delayed esophageal emptying, achalasia, hypocalcemia, and severe renal impairment with creatinine clearance below 30–35 mL/min, since they are cleared by the kidneys.

Side effects of BPs include upper gastrointestinal discomfort, indigestion, and heartburn. Oral BPs should be administered with a full glass of water, in the morning, on an empty stomach, and patients should remain upright for at least 30 min after the dose and delay eating for 30 min (with the exception of ibandronate, which requires 60 min). This procedure for administration is needed to improve bioavailability and mitigate gastrointestinal side effects. IV formulations can cause an acute phase reaction including fever and myalgias, and pretreatment with fluids and acetaminophen may prevent and reduce these symptoms [1]. Other adverse events include transient hypocalcemia, transient hypophosphatemia, myalgias, joint pain, back pain, headache, and dizziness. Rare but reported adverse effects include toxic epidermal necrosis and oropharyngeal ulceration [3]. BPs are associated with atypical femoral fractures (AFF) and osteonecrosis of jaw (ONJ), although these are rare events (5.9/100,000 person-years and 2/100,000 patient-years, respectively) [2]. It is important to weigh these rare complications against the significant benefits to reduce fracture risk. Adverse events from bisphosphonate therapy are further addressed in Chap. 12.

The FIT Long-term Extension Trial (FLEX) compared treatment duration with alendronate for 5 years versus 10 years [12]. The authors concluded that treatment with alendronate for 5 years was sufficient to maintain bone mass and decrease bone remodeling. The American Society for Bone and Mineral Research, the United States Preventive Services Task Force, and the American College of Physicians suggest consideration of a drug holiday after 3 years of treatment with intravenous zoledronic acid or

5 years with an oral BP. If there is high fracture risk, including patients with persistently low T-scores, previous major osteoporotic fractures, or fractures while on therapy, continuation of therapy for up to 10 years should be considered [2]. "Drug holidays" are further addressed in Chap. 15. Patients on oral bisphosphonates should be periodically monitored for treatment compliance.

Denosumab

Denosumab is the first biologic antiresorptive agent for osteoporosis. It is a fully human monoclonal antibody that inhibits receptor activator of nuclear factor-kappa B ligand (RANKL) to reduce bone resorption. RANKL is expressed on osteoblastic cells and binds to its receptor on RANK, present on the osteoclast surface and essential for osteoclast formation, activity, and survival [2].

Denosumab has been demonstrated to reduce vertebral, hip, and nonvertebral fractures in postmenopausal osteoporotic women. Denosumab has been approved by the FDA for the treatment of postmenopausal osteoporosis with high fracture risk, women with breast cancer receiving adjuvant aromatase inhibitor therapy, men with osteoporosis, men with prostate cancer receiving androgen deprivation therapy, and glucocorticoid-induced osteoporosis. The osteoporosis treatment dose is 60 mg subcutaneously every 6 months as a prefilled syringe administered by a healthcare professional. It is degraded independently of hepatic metabolism, with the serum concentration decreasing slowly over 3–5 months, and becoming undetectable after 6 months post dose in more than half of the recipients [13]. The American Association of Clinical Endocrinology and Endocrine Society guidelines recommend denosumab as a first-line treatment option [4, 5] (see Table 11.1).

The Fracture Reduction Evaluation of Denosumab in Osteoporosis Every 6 Months (FREEDOM Trial) was a randomized, placebo-controlled clinical trial which included 7868 postmenopausal women with osteoporosis [14]. Over a period of 3 years, denosumab significantly reduced the risk of vertebral fractures by 68%, nonvertebral fractures by 20%, and hip fractures by 40% compared to placebo. Denosumab reduces bone

Table 11.1 Antiresorptive agents, FDA-approved indications, and dosing

Antiresorptive agents	Indications	Treatment dosing
Bisphosphonates		
Alendronate	Osteoporosis in postmenopausal women and men Glucocorticoid-induced osteoporosis	10 mg PO daily or 70 mg PO weekly
Risedronate	Osteoporosis in postmenopausal women and men Glucocorticoid-induced osteoporosis	5 mg PO daily or 35 mg PO weekly or 150 mg PO monthly
Zoledronic acid	Osteoporosis in postmenopausal women and men Glucocorticoid-induced osteoporosis	5 mg IV annually
Ibandronate	Osteoporosis in postmenopausal women	2.5 mg PO daily or 150 mg PO monthly or 3 mg IV every 3 months
Denosumab	Osteoporosis in postmenopausal women and men Bone loss associated with aromatase inhibitor therapy in postmenopausal women with breast cancer Bone loss associated with androgen deprivation therapy in men with prostate cancer Glucocorticoid-induced osteoporosis	60 mg SC every 6 months
Selective estrogen receptor modulators		
Raloxifene	Osteoporosis in postmenopausal women	60 mg PO daily
Bazedoxifene-conjugated equine estrogen	Prevention of osteoporosis in postmenopausal women	20 mg/0.45 mg PO daily

Indications and doses taken from medication package insert

turnover markers, correlating with improvement in BMD at the lumbar spine and total hip. According to the open-label FREEDOM extension study through up to 10 years of denosumab treatment, there were continued increases in BMD without plateau, low fracture incidence compared with observed rates during the original trial, and overall low rates of adverse events [15].

Adverse events include AFF (0.8 per 10,000 patient-years), ONJ, skin infections, dermatological reactions, and hypocalcemia [13]. While denosumab therapy is not contraindicated in patients with decreased renal function, symptomatic hypocalcemia is a clinical concern in these patients, especially in those with creatinine clearance less than 30 mL/min and with end-stage renal disease on dialysis. Preexisting hypocalcemia is a contraindication for denosumab use and must be corrected before initiating treatment. Calcium levels should be monitored before each dose of denosumab, as well as within 2 weeks of the first dose in patients predisposed for hypocalcemia, such as patients with hypoparathyroidism, prior thyroid or parathyroid surgery, malabsorption syndromes, or small bowel resection [16].

Discontinuation of denosumab treatment is characterized by a transient increase in bone turnover markers and reversal of its favorable skeletal effects, referred to as "rebound phenomenon," with possible risk of multiple vertebral fractures. According to the European Calcified Tissue Society, fracture risk should be assessed after 3–5 years of treatment with denosumab. In individuals with high fracture risk, treatment should be continued for up to a total of 10 years or switched to alternative treatment, while those with low fracture risk may discontinue denosumab after 2.5 years. In either situation, therapy should be transitioned to an oral bisphosphonate for 12–24 months or zoledronic acid for 1–2 years to reduce or prevent the rebound increase in bone turnover, before giving a drug holiday [17]. The American Association of Clinical Endocrinology and Endocrine Society guidelines also recommend transitioning to another antiresorptive therapy after denosumab [4, 5]. Data suggest zoledronic acid may not be able to fully preserve bone density gains after discontinuation of denosumab [18]. The use of teriparatide following denosumab has been associated with bone loss at some skeletal sites, and therefore it may not be an effective sequential therapy after denosumab in high-risk patients [19].

Hormone Replacement Therapy (HRT)

Menopause is characterized by estrogen deficiency leading to bone loss and increased fracture risk. Hormone replacement therapy with combined estrogen and progesterone or estrogen alone has shown effectiveness in reducing vertebral and nonvertebral fractures in postmenopausal women. HRT is approved by the FDA for prevention of osteoporosis but not for treatment. Studies have shown that HRT is associated with increased risk of breast cancer, stroke, and coronary heart disease. However, it has been suggested that the route of administration and dosage of estrogen affects the severity of these adverse events. When compared to oral estrogen therapy, transdermal therapy has been associated with a reduced risk of atherosclerotic vascular disease. The risk benefit profile is also better when lower doses of estrogen are used. According to guidelines from the International Menopause Society, in women up to 60 years of age or within 10 years after menopause, benefits of HRT may outweigh the risks, and HRT can be used to relieve vasomotor symptoms of menopause along with BMD benefits. For women greater than 60 years of age or more than 10 years after menopause, initiation of HRT has to be individualized and is usually not recommended due to risks [20]. Endocrine Society guidelines suggest HRT can be used for therapy of osteoporosis in women <60 years and within 10 years of menopause with vasomotor and climacteric symptoms, without known contraindications, and for whom bisphosphonates or denosumab are not appropriate [5].

Selective Estrogen Receptor Modulators (SERMs)

Selective estrogen receptor modulators (SERMs) have estrogen-agonist effects on bone and estrogen-antagonist effects in breast tissue, thereby affecting bone homeostasis by downregulating osteoclast activity and reducing bone resorption. While SERMs can improve bone density and decrease vertebral fracture risk in postmenopausal osteoporosis, they have opposite effects in premenopausal women as they compete with estrogen and are weaker agonists than estrogen. The SERM class includes tamoxifen, raloxifene, lasofoxifene, and bazedoxifene. Raloxifene has been FDA approved for treatment of postmenopausal osteoporosis and bazedoxifene-conjugated estrogen approved for prevention of postmenopausal osteoporosis. SERMs are primarily used in young postmenopausal women and are particularly recommended if there is a family history of invasive breast cancer, since their use reduces the incidence of breast cancer. They can maintain BMD and help reduce incidence of vertebral fractures, but do not reduce hip or nonvertebral fractures. Common side effects include hot flashes and atrophic vaginitis. SERMs have been associated with a higher risk of venous thromboembolism, including deep vein thrombosis, pulmonary embolism, and stroke [21] (Table 11.1).

Outcome

Risk factors for osteoporosis in our patient included postmenopausal status, vitamin D deficiency, and carbamazepine use. After discussion of risks and benefits, she was most interested in therapy with denosumab. She has started treatment with denosumab every 6 months and is due for repeat DXA scan after 2 years of treatment to help determine the treatment course. She is aware of the need to transition to a bisphosphonate prior to a "drug holiday" from treatment.

Clinical Pearls/Pitfalls
- Antiresorptive agents include bisphosphonates, denosumab, hormone replacement therapy, and selective estrogen receptor modulators (SERMs).
- Bisphosphonates (alendronate, risedronate, and zoledronic acid) and denosumab have demonstrated benefit against vertebral, hip, and nonvertebral fractures and are

FDA approved for treatment of postmenopausal osteo-porosis in women, osteoporosis in men, and for gluco-corticoid-induced osteoporosis.
- Adverse events of bisphosphonates and denosumab include transient hypocalcemia, atypical femoral fractures, and osteonecrosis of the jaw.
- Drug holidays are suggested with bisphosphonate therapy.
- Discontinuation of denosumab results in "rebound phenomenon," characterized by the reversal of favorable skeletal effects. Denosumab therapy should be followed with a bisphosphonate.
- Hormone replacement therapy can be used for osteoporosis in postmenopausal women, but it is not recommended as a first-line treatment option.
- SERMs are used in postmenopausal women of young age and particularly recommended in those with a family history of invasive breast cancer.

References

1. Tu KN, Lie JD, Wan CKV, Cameron M, Austel AG, et al. Osteoporosis: a review of treatment options. P T. 2018;43(2):92–104.
2. Akkawi I, Zmerly H. Osteoporosis: current concepts. Joints. 2018;6(2):122–7.
3. Eriksen EF, Díez-Pérez A, Boonen S. Update on long-term treatment with bisphosphonates for postmenopausal osteoporosis: a systematic review. Bone. 2014;58:126–35.
4. Camacho PM, Petak SM, Binkley N, Diab DL, Eldeiry LS, et al. American Association of Clinical Endocrinologists/American College of Endocrinology Clinical Practice Guidelines for the diagnosis and treatment of postmenopausal osteoporosis-2020 update. Endocr Pract. 2020;26(Suppl 1):1–46.
5. Eastell R, Rosen CJ, Black DM, Cheung AM, Murad MH, Shoback D. Pharmacological management of osteoporosis in postmenopausal women: an Endocrine Society clinical practice guideline. J Clin Endocrinol Metab. 2019;104(5):1595–622.

6. Black DM, Thompson DE, Bauer DC, Ensrud K, Musliner T, et al. Fracture risk reduction with alendronate in women with osteoporosis: the Fracture Intervention Trial. FIT Research Group. J Clin Endocrinol Metab. 2000;85(11):4118–24.
7. Wells GA, Cranney A, Peterson J, Boucher M, Shea B, Robinson V, Coyle D, Tugwell P. Alendronate for the primary and secondary prevention of osteoporotic fractures in postmenopausal women. Cochrane Database Syst Rev. 2008;(1):CD001155.
8. Cranney A, Tugwell P, Adachi J, Weaver B, Zytaruk N, et al. Meta-analyses of therapies for postmenopausal osteoporosis. III. Meta-analysis of risedronate for the treatment of postmenopausal osteoporosis. Endocr Rev. 2002;23(4):517.
9. Reid DM, Hosking D, Kendler D, Brandi ML, Wark JD, et al. A comparison of the effect of alendronate and risedronate on bone mineral density in postmenopausal women with osteoporosis: 24-month results from FACTS-International. Int J Clin Pract. 2008;62(4):575–84.
10. Black DM, Delmas PD, Eastell R, Reid IR, Boonen S, et al. Once-yearly zoledronic acid for treatment of postmenopausal osteoporosis. N Engl J Med. 2007;356:1809–22.
11. Räkel A, Boucher A, Ste-Marie LG. Role of zoledronic acid in the prevention and treatment of osteoporosis. Clin Interv Aging. 2011;6:89–99.
12. Black DM, Schwartz AV, Ensrud KE, Cauley JA, Levis S, et al. Effects of continuing or stopping alendronate after 5 years of treatment: the Fracture Intervention Trial Long-term Extension (FLEX): a randomized trial. JAMA. 2006;296(24):2927–38.
13. Deeks ED. Denosumab: a review in postmenopausal osteoporosis. Drugs Aging. 2018;35(2):163–73.
14. Cummings SR, San Martin J, McClung MR, Siris ES, Eastell R, et al. Denosumab for prevention of fractures in postmenopausal women with osteoporosis. N Engl J Med. 2009;361(8):756–65.
15. Bone HG, Wagman RB, Brandi ML, Brown JP, Chapurlat R, et al. 10 years of denosumab treatment in postmenopausal women with osteoporosis: results from the phase 3 randomised FREEDOM trial and open-label extension. Lancet Diabetes Endocrinol. 2017;5(7):513–23.
16. Lewiecki EM. New and emerging concepts in the use of denosumab for the treatment of osteoporosis. Ther Adv Musculoskelet Dis. 2018;10(11):209–23.
17. Tsourdi E, Zillikens MC, Meier C, Body JJ, Gonzalez Rodriguez E, et al. Fracture risk and management of discontinuation of denosumab therapy: a systematic review and position statement by ECTS. J Clin Endocrinol Metab. 2020:dgaa756. https://doi.org/10.1210/clinem/dgaa756. Online ahead of print.
18. Sølling AS, Harsløf T, Langdahl B. Treatment with zoledronate subsequent to denosumab in osteoporosis: a randomized trial. J Bone Miner Res. 2020;35(10):1858–70.

19. Leder BZ, Tsai JN, Uihlein AV, et al. Denosumab and teriparatide transitions in postmenopausal osteoporosis (the DATA-switch study): extension of a randomised controlled trial. Lancet. 2015;386:1147–55.
20. Baber RJ, Panay N, Fenton A, IMS Writing Group. 2016 IMS recommendations on women's midlife health and menopause hormone therapy. Climacteric. 2016;19(2):109–50.
21. An KC. Selective estrogen receptor modulators. Asian Spine J. 2016;10(4):787–91.

Adverse Effects of Antiresorptive Therapy

12

Sumeet Jain and Pauline Camacho

Case Presentation

A 68-year-old man with a history of metastatic oral squamous cell cancer, type 2 diabetes, and tobacco abuse presented for evaluation of osteoporosis. He was diagnosed with a pathologic lumbar compression fracture after developing sharp back pain after bending down to pick up a box. DXA scan showed osteoporosis with T score of −2.6 and BMD of 0.856 g/cm^2 at the L spine. He was treated with monthly zoledronic acid infusions by his oncologist. He declined to quit smoking. After four zoledronic acid infusions, he saw his dentist and had a dental extraction. The dental extraction site was complicated by an abscess with exposed bone 1 week later. He was diagnosed with stage 2 osteonecrosis of the jaw similar to Fig. 12.1. He was treated with incision and drainage and antibiotics. His zoledronic acid was held, and osteoporosis was treated supportively with nutritional supplementation, fall avoid-

S. Jain (✉)
Division of Endocrinology, Rush University Medical Center,
Chicago, IL, USA
e-mail: Sumeet_Jain@rush.edu

P. Camacho
Division of Endocrinology, Loyola University Osteoporosis and
Metabolic Bone Disease Center, Loyola University Medical Center,
Maywood, IL, USA

© The Author(s), under exclusive license to Springer Nature
Switzerland AG 2021
N. E. Cusano (ed.), *Osteoporosis*,
https://doi.org/10.1007/978-3-030-83951-2_12

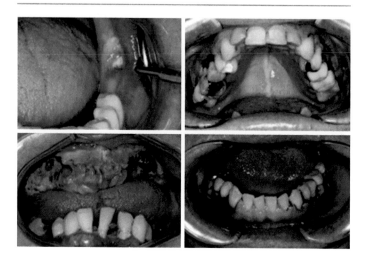

Fig. 12.1 Stages of osteonecrosis of the jaw. Top left picture with stage 1 osteonecrosis of the jaw with asymptomatic exposed bone without infection. Right-sided pictures with stage 2 osteonecrosis of the jaw with exposed bone and associated infection, bleeding, swelling, pain, and halitosis at preexisting areas of periodontitis. Bottom left picture with stage 3 osteonecrosis of the jaw with large areas of bone exposure, pus exudation, and a chronic oroantral fistula. (Adapted from Otto et al. [1])

ance, and weight-bearing exercise. He had delayed healing but achieved complete surgical healing 6 months later.

Background

Osteonecrosis of the jaw is defined as an area of exposed bone in the maxillofacial region that does not heal within 8 weeks after identification by a healthcare provider, in a patient who has received antiresorptive therapy with no history of radiation to the jaw [2]. Bisphosphonate-related osteonecrosis of the jaw has been reported with both bisphosphonate and denosumab treatment. It is exceedingly rare in patients treated for osteoporosis with an incidence of less than 1 event in 100,000 patient years for oral bisphosphonates, less than 1 event in 10,000 patient years for IV bisphosphonates, and less than 1 event in 10,000 patient years for denosumab. Over 90% of reported cases have been associated with cancer with an incidence of 0–12,222 events in 100,000 patient years for IV bisphosphonates and 0 to 2316 events in 100,000 patient years for denosumab in patients treated for cancer [2].

Risk Factors

- Smoking
- Poor dental hygiene or ill-fitting dentures
- Cancer with higher of more frequent dosing
- Extended duration of antiresorptive therapy
- Invasive dental work
- Diabetes mellitus
- Antiangiogenic medications (anti-VEGF monoclonal antibodies, tyrosine kinase inhibitors, and mTOR inhibitors) [3]
- Steroids
- Illicit drug use [4]

Clinical Pearls

- Osteonecrosis of the jaw is exceedingly rare when used for osteoporosis treatment.
- Osteonecrosis of the jaw is a significant clinical consideration when used for cancer treatment.
- Limit above modifiable risk factors when using antiresorptive therapy.
- Complete invasive dental therapies prior to start of antiresorptive therapy. Due to the long half-life of bisphosphonates and risk of rebound fractures with denosumab discontinuation, holding antiresorptive medications is not generally recommended in patients undergoing dental procedures already on antiresorptive treatment.

- Symptoms: Exposed bone, fistula, edema, purulence, perioral paresthesia or pain, loose teeth, halitosis.
- Treatment (based on severity): Improving oral hygiene, topical antibiotic mouth rinses, systemic antibiotics, surgical removal of necrotic bone, and jaw reconstruction.

Case Presentation

A 72-year-old woman with history of postmenopausal osteoporosis presented to the hospital with a left leg fracture after collapsing without trauma while walking. She had noted nonspecific dull bilateral groin pain for 4 months prior to her fracture. She was diagnosed with osteoporosis on a screening DXA at age 60 and was started on weekly alendronate. She was not started on a bisphosphonate holiday, and she had been strictly adherent with taking weekly alendronate for the past 12 years. X-ray of the left femur showed a transverse midshaft femoral diaphysis fracture with thickened bone cortices similar to Fig. 12.2b. X-ray of the right femur showed a translucent lucency of the lateral femoral cortex perpendicular to the femoral surface consistent with an impending atypical femur fracture similar to Fig. 12.2a. Her left femur was surgically stabilized, and a prophylactic intramedullary rod was placed in her right femur. Bisphosphonate therapy was stopped.

Background

An atypical femur fracture is a fracture on the femoral diaphysis distal to the lesser trochanter and proximal to the supracondylar flare. It is diagnosed with four out of five major features: minimal or no associated trauma, mostly transverse fracture line with origination at the lateral cortex, noncomminuted or minimally comminuted fracture (without multiple bone fragments), medial spike when fracture is complete, and localized periosteal or endosteal thickening of the lateral cortex. Common minor associated features not required for diagnosis include increased femoral

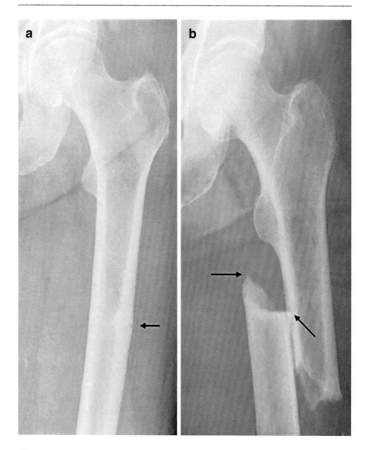

Fig. 12.2 (**a**) Impending atypical femoral fracture with arrow pointing at localized periosteal thickening at the lateral cortex. (**b**) Complete midshaft atypical femoral fracture with left arrow pointing at the medial spike and right arrow pointing at the transverse lateral cortex fracture origin. (Adapted from Nguyen et al. [5])

diaphysis cortical thickness, unilateral or bilateral prodromal dull pain in the groin or thigh, bilateral involvement, and delayed fracture healing [6].

Atypical femur fractures are most commonly associated with bisphosphonate therapy though they have also been seen with

other antiresorptive medications including denosumab and romosozumab. Atypical femur fractures are a particularly distressing
side effect for patients because they occur as a complication of a
medication taken to prevent fractures. However, the benefits of
bisphosphonate therapy for fractures are magnitudes larger than
the harms. In one analysis of bisphosphonate treatment for
3 years, approximately 1200 fractures including 130 devastating
typical femur fractures were prevented for every 1 atypical femur
fracture caused by bisphosphonate therapy [7, 8]. The risk of
atypical femur fractures is higher in Asian American women but
still has greater benefit than harm with 13.8 fractures including
4.6 typical hip fractures prevented for every 1 atypical femur fracture caused by 5 years of bisphosphonate therapy [9].

Risk Factors

- Antiresorptive medications
- Longer duration of antiresorptive medication use
- Asian ethnicity (in North American and European studies)
- Hypophosphatasia
- Osteomalacia
- Femur geometry with increased femoral bowing
- Glucocorticoids
- Genetics [8]

Clinical Pearls

- Atypical femur fractures are extremely rare compared to typical femur fractures.
- Ask about nonspecific prodromal thigh or groin pain for
  patients on antiresorptive therapy.
- Look at your own DXA images, not just reports. Evaluate for
  localized lateral periosteal breaking (periosteal thickening)
  and transverse lucency at the lateral femoral cortex. Refer for

prophylactic fixation if impending atypical femoral fracture present.

- Consider bisphosphonate holiday for oral bisphosphonates after 5 years of therapy if fracture risk is no longer high and after 10 years if patient remains at high fracture risk. Consider bisphosphonate holiday for intravenous zoledronic acid after 3 years of therapy if fracture risk is no longer high and after 6 years if patient remains at high fracture risk [10].
- Atypical femur fractures are frequently bilateral so image the contralateral femur when an atypical femur fracture occurs.
- Delayed healing is common after atypical femur fractures.
- Imaging: X-ray appearance in Fig. 12.2. If high clinical suspicion despite negative X-ray, MRI may show periosteal or adjacent bone marrow inflammation/edema and bone scintigraphy may show increased uptake and local periosteal stress reaction.
- Symptoms: Weeks to months of nonspecific thigh or groin pain.
- Treatment: Discontinue antiresorptive therapy, supplement calcium and vitamin D, reduce weight bearing for 2–3 months with crutches or a walker (for impending fractures), surgical intramedullary fixation, and consider anabolic treatment with teriparatide or abaloparatide.

Case Presentation

An 80-year-old woman with a history of postmenopausal osteoporosis and vitamin D deficiency was treated with her first zoledronic acid infusion. She did not start recommended vitamin D or calcium supplementation prior to her infusion. Two days after the infusion, she called the clinic with concerns she was having fevers, myalgias, photophobia, and decreased visual acuity in her left eye. She was started on acetaminophen treatment and was evaluated by an ophthalmologist who diagnosed her with uveitis and started her on topical ophthalmic corticosteroids. Her symptoms resolved 1 week after her infusion. She started her vitamin supplements and was rechallenged with zoledronic acid 1 year later with no side effects.

Background

Acute phase reactions after bisphosphonate therapy are the most common side effect of IV bisphosphonate therapy. They are thought to be caused by an inflammatory cascade release related to T-cell activation. These reactions occur within 3 days of bisphosphonate infusion and may include flu-like symptoms like fever, chills, headache, and malaise; musculoskeletal symptoms like myalgias and arthralgias; gastrointestinal symptoms like nausea and anorexia; and inflammatory eye disease symptoms like uveitis, scleritis, and iritis. In the HORIZON-Pivotal fracture trial for zoledronic acid, 30% more patients in the zoledronic acid arm had an infusion acute phase reaction than in the placebo arm [11]. Symptoms are mostly mild and generally resolve without treatment in 3–5 days. Patients generally do not have infusion reactions with subsequent infusions with 7% incidence at the second infusion and 3% incidence at the third infusion of zoledronic acid [11]. Oral bisphosphonates are associated with less frequent (5.6% incidence in a retrospective study) and milder acute phase reactions [12]. Higher vitamin D levels at time of infusion decrease acute phase reactions [13].

Inflammatory eye disease after bisphosphonate therapy is rare and occurs in 0.6–1.1% of patients treated with IV bisphosphonates and much lower rates for patients treated with oral bisphosphonates [13, 14]. Ocular involvement can be either unilateral or bilateral. It is commonly but not always associated with other acute phase reaction symptoms described above. It is mostly easily treated within 4 weeks with topical corticosteroids, but some cases do require systemic corticosteroids or procedural intervention. It is important for endocrinologists and ophthalmologists to know about bisphosphonate-related inflammatory eye disease to avoid unnecessary expensive testing and antibiotic or antiviral treatments.

Risk Factors

- Nonsteroidal anti-inflammatory (NSAID) use
- Vitamin D less than 30 ng/mL (75 nmol/L) [13]
- Initial antiresorptive treatment

Clinical Pearls

- Supplement vitamin D and calcium to normal levels before starting antiresorptive treatment.
- Pretreat patients with acetaminophen and increased water intake prior to IV bisphosphonate infusion.
- Acute phase reactions are not an absolute contraindication to future bisphosphonate infusion since they occur less frequently with subsequent infusions.
- Symptoms: Fevers, myalgias, arthralgias, malaise, photophobia, and decreased visual acuity.
- Treatment: Acetaminophen, increased water intake, vitamin D and calcium supplementation, topical or systemic corticosteroids, and ophthalmology referral for inflammatory eye disease.

Case Presentation

An 85-year-old woman with chronic kidney disease (CKD) stage 3B and multivessel coronary artery disease with previous coronary artery bypass grafting was recently diagnosed with postmenopausal osteoporosis after she was found to have a nontraumatic vertebral compression fracture. Secondary osteoporosis evaluation was unremarkable. She was unable to be started on anabolic therapy since she is unable to give herself daily teriparatide or abaloparatide injections with arthritis in her hands, and she declines romosozumab therapy due to her cardiovascular history. She declines denosumab therapy because she travels frequently, and she does not think she can be available for every 6-month injections. Her eGFR is 38 mL/min which has been confirmed with 24-h urine creatinine and blood cystatin C measurement. She would like to have osteoporosis treatment with IV zoledronic acid, but she wants to know if there is any risk of progression of chronic kidney disease with bisphosphonate treatment.

Background

Bisphosphonate use is generally contraindicated in CKD stage 4 when eGFR is <30 mL/min due to concerns for nephrotoxicity. For zoledronic acid and alendronate, the threshold is <35 mL/min. Approximately 50–60% of bisphosphonate therapy is excreted by the kidneys, and the rest is taken up by the bone [15]. Case reports of acute tubular necrosis on IV bisphosphonate therapy have been mostly reported in the multiple myeloma population when patients receive high-dose IV bisphosphonates at frequent intervals. The renal safety of both PO and IV bisphosphonates has previously been shown in multiple randomized controlled trials including the HORIZON-Pivotal trial for zoledronic acid that showed no renal harm compared to placebo after 3 years of therapy. A recent observational study from the UK and Spain found a 14% increased relative risk for CKD progression in patients treated with bisphosphonates with eGFR < 45 mL/min including patients with CKD 3B, CKD4, and CKD 5 [16]. Approximately two-thirds of their cohort had eGFR of 35–45 suggesting there may be some modest long-term progression of CKD related to bisphosphonate use in CKD stage 3B.

Risk Factors

- NSAID use
- Poor hydration with bisphosphonate infusions
- Diuretics
- CKD 4 with eGFR < 30 mL/min and possibly CKD 3B with eGFR < 45 mL/min

- Higher bisphosphonate dose
- Shorter bisphosphonate infusion duration
- Other nephrotoxic medications

Clinical Pearls

- Reassess eGFR prior to each bisphosphonate infusion.
- Avoid nephrotoxins including NSAIDs with bisphosphonate use.
- Advise oral hydration with bisphosphonate infusions.
- Give bisphosphonates as longer infusions when used with impaired kidney function.
- Balance mortality and quality of life benefits from bisphosphonate therapy with possible modest CKD progression risk in CKD stage 3B and lower.

Case Presentation

A 64-year-old man with a 50-pack-year smoking history, alcohol dependence, and osteoarthritis on ibuprofen was found to have osteoporosis on a screening DXA scan. He had no history of fractures and has normal kidney function so he was started on alendronate 70 mg once a week. He works long hours and drinks three cups of coffee per day. One month later, he called the office stating that he is getting epigastric pain after taking his alendronate pill. Upon further discussion, he notes that he had years of dyspepsia symptoms prior to starting alendronate therapy, but symptoms have worsened in the past month. Alendronate was stopped, and he had an upper endoscopy with a gastroenterologist that found erosive esophagitis. He was counseled on tobacco and alcohol cessation, NSAID avoidance, counseled on dietary changes, and started on a proton pump inhibitor (PPI) for gastroesophageal reflux disease (GERD). He was transitioned to yearly zoledronic acid infusions for his osteoporosis. His epigastric pain resolved 3 months later.

Background

Upper gastrointestinal (GI) side effects are the most common cause of oral bisphosphonate discontinuation by patients. GI side effects account for up to 40% of oral bisphosphonate discontinuation [17]. Oral bisphosphonates can contribute to nausea, emesis, dyspepsia, abdominal pain, erosive esophagitis, gastritis, and duodenitis. These symptoms are thought to be mediated by direct topical irritation. They may also displace phospholipids from the GI mucosal gel layer and impair mucosal healing [18]. GI mucosal irritation has been confirmed on endoscopic studies, but interestingly increased GI adverse events from oral bisphosphonates have not been shown in placebo-controlled randomized controlled trials like the FIT trial for alendronate or the VERT trial for risedronate [18, 19]. They also were not seen in a large meta-analysis of 42 randomized controlled trials and 40,000 participants [18]. This suggests there may be some bias of patients and physicians toward reporting GI symptoms. A case control study of mostly older men did find a twofold increase in Barrett's esophagus in veterans on bisphosphonate therapy, but that association was only significant in patients with active GERD symptoms [20]. Older studies that were done before the advent of weekly oral bisphosphonate dosing and before guidance to remain upright for 30 min after oral bisphosphonate ingestion tended to have higher rates of GI adverse events than more recent studies.

Risk Factors

- NSAID use
- Active GERD symptoms
- GI motility disorders
- Esophageal strictures

Clinical Pearls

- Advise patient to sit up or stand up for 30 min after taking a bisphosphonate pill with a full glass of water.

- For patients with uncontrolled GERD, intravenous zoledronic acid therapy is preferred over oral bisphosphonate therapy.
- Avoid oral bisphosphonates in patients with Barrett's esophagus, active esophagitis, or active GERD symptoms.
- Work on controlling GERD prior to starting oral bisphosphonate therapy. Modifiable GERD risk factors include coffee, tea, soda, chocolate, alcohol, tobacco, eating while recumbent, eating within 2 h of sleeping, and obesity.
- PPI therapy may be considered for mild GERD symptoms for patients prescribed oral bisphosphonates, though GI benefits of PPIs must be weighed against their adverse effects on bone and kidney health in large population studies.
- Symptoms: Dyspepsia, abdominal pain, chest pain, nausea, and emesis.
- Treatment: Address modifiable GERD risk factors, switch to intravenous or injection osteoporosis therapy if GERD is unable to be controlled.

References

1. Otto S, Pautke C, Van den Wyngaert T, Niepel D, Schiødt M. Medication-related osteonecrosis of the jaw: prevention, diagnosis and management in patients with cancer and bone metastases. Cancer Treat Rev. 2018;69:177–87.
2. Khan A, Morrison A, Hanley D, Felsenberg D, McCauley L, O'Ryan F, et al. Diagnosis and management of osteonecrosis of the jaw: a systematic review and international consensus. J Bone Miner Res. 2014;30(1):3–23.
3. Pimolbutr K, Porter S, Fedele S. Osteonecrosis of the jaw associated with antiangiogenics in antiresorptive-naïve patient: a comprehensive review of the literature. Biomed Res Int. 2018;2018:1–14.
4. Sacco R, Ball R, Barry E, Akintola O. The role of illicit drugs in developing medication-related osteonecrosis (MRONJ): a systematic review. Br J Oral Maxillofac Surg. 2021;59(4):398–406.
5. Nguyen H, Milat F, Ebeling P. A new contralateral atypical femoral fracture despite sequential therapy with teriparatide and strontium ranelate. Bone Rep. 2017;6:34–7.
6. Shane E, Burr D, Abrahamsen B, Adler R, Brown T, Cheung A, et al. Atypical subtrochanteric and diaphyseal femoral fractures: second report of a task force of the American Society for Bone and Mineral Research. J Bone Miner Res. 2013;29(1):1–23.

7. Black D, Rosen C. Postmenopausal osteoporosis. N Engl J Med. 2016;374(3):254–62.

8. Black D, Abrahamsen B, Bouxsein M, Einhorn T, Napoli N. Atypical femur fractures: review of epidemiology, relationship to bisphosphonates, prevention, and clinical management. Endocr Rev. 2018;40(2):333–68.

9. Black D, Geiger E, Eastell R, Vittinghoff E, Li B, Ryan D, et al. Atypical femur fracture risk versus fragility fracture prevention with bisphosphonates. N Engl J Med. 2020;383(8):743–53.

10. Camacho P, Petak S, Binkley N, Diab D, Eldeiry L, Farooki A, et al. American Association of Clinical Endocrinologists/American College of Endocrinology Clinical Practice Guidelines for the diagnosis and treatment of postmenopausal osteoporosis—2020 update. Endocr Pract. 2020;26:1–46.

11. Reid I, Gamble G, Mesenbrink P, Lakatos P, Black D. Characterization of and risk factors for the acute-phase response after zoledronic acid. J Clin Endocrinol Metabol. 2010;95(9):4380–7.

12. Lim S, Bolster M. What can we do about musculoskeletal pain from bisphosphonates? Cleve Clin J Med. 2018;85(9):675–8.

13. Crotti C, Watts N, De Santis M, Ceribelli A, Fabbriciani G, Cavaciocchi F, et al. Acute phase reactions after zoledronic acid infusion: protective role of 25-hydroxyvitamin D and previous oral bisphosphonate therapy. Endocr Pract. 2018;24(5):405–10.

14. Tian Y, Wang R, Liu L, Ma C, Lu Q, Yin F. Acute bilateral uveitis and right macular edema induced by a single infusion of zoledronic acid for the treatment of postmenopausal osteoporosis as a substitution for oral alendronate: a case report. BMC Musculoskelet Disord. 2016;17(1):72.

15. Khosla S, Bilezikian J, Dempster D, Lewiecki E, Miller P, Neer R, et al. Benefits and risks of bisphosphonate therapy for osteoporosis. J Clin Endocrinol Metabol. 2012;97(7):2272–82.

16. Robinson D, Ali M, Pallares N, Tebé C, Elhussein L, Abrahamsen B, et al. Safety of oral bisphosphonates in moderate-to-severe chronic kidney disease: a binational cohort analysis. J Bone Miner Res. 2021;36(5):820–32.

17. Goldshtein I, Rouach V, Shamir-Stein N, Yu J, Chodick G. Role of side effects, physician involvement, and patient perception in non-adherence with oral bisphosphonates. Adv Ther. 2016;33(8):1374–84.

18. Dömötör Z, Vörhendi N, Hanák L, Hegyi P, Kiss S, Csiki E, et al. Oral treatment with bisphosphonates of osteoporosis does not increase the risk of severe gastrointestinal side effects: a meta-analysis of randomized controlled trials. Front Endocrinol. 2020;11:573976.

19. Lanza F. Gastrointestinal adverse effects of bisphosphonates. Treat Endocrinol. 2002;1(1):37–43.

20. Lin D, Kramer J, Ramsey D, Alsarraj A, Verstovsek G, Rugge M, et al. Oral bisphosphonates and the risk of Barrett's esophagus: case–control analysis of US veterans. Am J Gastroenterol. 2013;108(10):1576–83.

PTH and PTHrP Analogs

Natalie E. Cusano

Case Presentation

A 65-year-old woman was referred for evaluation of recently diagnosed osteoporosis. She sustained a left distal radius fracture 2 months prior in a fall from standing height onto a sidewalk. Subsequent bone density testing was significant for T-scores of −3.5 at the lumbar spine, −3.1 at the femoral neck, and −2.8 at the total hip. She had a history of thalassemia trait but no other significant past medical history and no history of radiation exposure. She had no previous personal history of fracture. Her mother had a history of osteoporosis, but there was no parental history of hip fracture. She had two servings of dairy per day and was taking a multivitamin with 300 mg of calcium and 1000 IU of vitamin D. She had no history of tobacco use and drank alcohol rarely. Her body mass index was 22 kg/m^2, and physical examination was otherwise unremarkable. Metabolic evaluation for secondary causes of bone loss was unremarkable, including normal serum calcium, PTH, and alkaline phosphatase levels. She was very interested in osteoanabolic therapy when discussed at the time of her visit.

N. E. Cusano (✉)
Division of Endocrinology, Lenox Hill Hospital, New York, NY, USA
e-mail: ncusano@northwell.edu

© The Author(s), under exclusive license to Springer Nature Switzerland AG 2021
N. E. Cusano (ed.), *Osteoporosis*,
https://doi.org/10.1007/978-3-030-83951-2_13

Assessment and Diagnosis

In contrast to antiresorptive agents, osteoanabolic therapies directly stimulate bone formation, improving not only bone mass but also bone microstructure [1]. Because bone formation and bone resorption are tightly coupled processes, osteoanabolic therapy will eventually stimulate bone resorption as well. The period of time when bone formation is greater than resorption is termed the anabolic window (Fig. 13.1) [2].

Parathyroid hormone has both anabolic and catabolic effects on bone. In patients with primary hyperparathyroidism, chronically elevated PTH levels have been associated with bone loss and increased fracture risk. In contrast, when PTH is given intermittently, with PTH levels rising and falling over a short period of time,

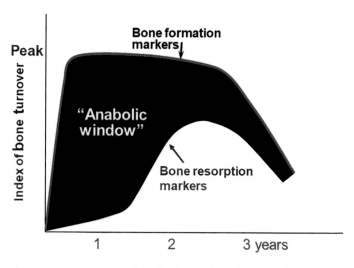

Fig. 13.1 Demonstration of the "anabolic window" concept that bone formation is first stimulated by an osteoanabolic agent followed by an increase in bone resorption [2]

there can be exuberant bone formation. The anabolic effects of PTH on bone are likely multifactorial, including pathways involving Wnt, Runx2, and insulin-like growth factor-1 (IGF-1) [1].

Teriparatide [PTH(1–34)] is the first 34 amino acids of the 84 amino acid parathyroid hormone protein. Abaloparatide is a functional optimization of parathyroid hormone-related peptide (PTHrP) based on amino acid substitutions between residues 22 and 34 [3].

Osteoanabolic therapy with teriparatide was approved by the Food and Drug Administration in 2002 for postmenopausal women and men at high risk for fracture and in 2009 for women and men with glucocorticoid-induced osteoporosis at high risk for fracture [4]. Per the approval, patients at high risk for fracture were defined as those who had experienced an osteoporotic fracture or patients with multiple risk factors for fracture. Teriparatide is used at a dose of 20 μg subcutaneously (SC) daily, typically for up to 24 months.

Abaloparatide was approved by the FDA in 2017 for treatment of osteoporosis in postmenopausal women at high risk for fracture or patients who have failed or are intolerant to other available osteoporosis therapy [5]. Abaloparatide is used at a dose of 80 μg SC daily, typically for up to 18 months.

The definitions of high fracture risk may differ, although there is general consensus encompassing patients who have already suffered a fracture. Hodsman and colleagues defined this group as patients with preexisting fractures, patients with a T-score of −3.5 or lower, and/or an unsatisfactory response to antiresorptive therapy [6]. Guidelines from the American Association of Clinical Endocrinology (AACE) [7] and Endocrine Society [8] recommend osteoanabolic therapy as first-line treatment for patients who are at very high risk for fracture. The AACE guidelines defined very high risk patients as patients with a fracture within 12 months, fractures while on approved osteoporosis therapy, multiple fractures, fractures while on drugs causing skeletal harm (e.g., glucocorticoids), very low T-score (<−3.0), high risk for falls or injurious falls, and very high fracture probability by FRAX (major osteoporotic fracture risk >30%, hip fracture >4.5%). Endocrine Society guidelines state very high risk patients include those with severe or multiple vertebral fractures.

In animal toxicity studies, male and female rats treated with PTH or PTH analogs were at an increased risk of osteosarcoma; however, this increased risk was not seen in monkeys [4]. Osteoanabolic therapy is contraindicated in patients at increased risk for osteosarcoma, including patients with open epiphyses, Paget's disease of bone or unexplained elevations of alkaline phosphatase, or prior external beam radiation therapy involving the skeleton.

Management

Osteoanabolic agents have been demonstrated to stimulate bone formation, improve bone density, and decrease vertebral and non-vertebral fracture risk. The pivotal trial leading to approval of teriparatide was a randomized, multicenter, double-blind, placebo-controlled trial in postmenopausal women that demonstrated an increase in bone density at the lumbar spine of +9.7% ($p < 0.001$) in the teriparatide 20 µg arm compared to placebo, +2.8% at the femoral neck ($p < 0.001$), and +2.6% at the total hip ($p < 0.001$) at a mean of 18 months of therapy [8]. There were relative risk reductions of 0.35 (95% CI, 0.22–0.55) for vertebral fracture and 0.47 (95% CI, 0.25–0.88) for nonvertebral fracture with the teriparatide 20 µg dose. Men were subsequently demonstrated to have similar improvements in bone density [9].

Teriparatide was compared to alendronate 10 mg PO daily in a randomized, multicenter, double-blind trial for women and men with glucocorticoid-induced osteoporosis [10]. There were significantly greater increases in bone density at the lumbar spine in the teriparatide versus alendronate group (+7.2% vs. 3.4%; $p < 0.001$) and at the total hip (3.8% vs. 2.4%; $p = 0.005$) at 18 months. Morphometric vertebral fractures were noted in 0.6% of patients in the teriparatide arm versus 6.1% in the alendronate arm ($p = 0.004$); there were no differences between groups in non-vertebral fractures. The study was extended for an additional 18 months, with findings that continued to demonstrate greater gains in bone density in the teriparatide over the alendronate arms

(11.0% vs. 5.3% at the lumbar spine; $p < 0.001$) as well as a decrease in fracture incidence (1.7% vs. 7.7%; $p = 0.007$) [11].

The pivotal trial leading to approval of abaloparatide was the Abaloparatide Comparator Trial in Vertebral Endpoints (ACTIVE), a randomized, multicenter, double-blind, placebo-controlled, active comparator (unblinded), 18-month trial in post-menopausal women with three arms: abaloparatide 80 μg SC daily, placebo SC, or teriparatide 20 μg SC daily [12]. Bone density at the lumbar spine increased similarly between the abaloparatide and teriparatide groups (+11.2% vs. +10.5%) and significantly greater than placebo (+0.63%; $p < 0.05$ compared to abaloparatide and teriparatide). Bone density at the femoral neck increased to a greater extent in the abaloparatide arm (+3.6%) compared to teriparatide (+2.7%; $p < 0.05$) and placebo (−0.43%; $p < 0.05$). Bone density at the total hip also increased to a greater extent in the abaloparatide arm (+4.2%) compared to teriparatide (+3.3%; $p < 0.05$) and placebo (−0.10%; $p < 0.05$). Vertebral fractures were similarly decreased in the abaloparatide (RR 0.14, 0.05–0.39) and teriparatide (0.20, 0.08–0.47) arms compared to placebo ($p < 0.001$ for both). Major osteoporotic fractures were decreased in the abaloparatide arm compared to both the teriparatide (HR 0.45 for abaloparatide versus teriparatide, 0.21–0.95; $p = 0.03$) and placebo groups (HR 0.30 for abaloparatide versus placebo, 0.15–0.61 $p < 0.001$).

Bone density at the spine and hip sites declines rapidly after osteoanabolic therapy is discontinued, and it is important to note that osteoanabolic therapy must be followed by antiresorptive therapy so that patients do not lose the bone that was gained [13].

Studies have investigated the combination of an antiresorptive and teriparatide therapy together. Oral or intravenous bisphosphonate therapy in combination with teriparatide has not been demonstrated to have significant additive effects, and in fact bisphosphonate therapy may attenuate the effect of teriparatide [14–16]. Combination of denosumab and teriparatide therapy was shown to increase bone density more than either agent alone; however, fracture data are not available [17]. It should be noted that combination therapy has not been approved.

The timing of therapy appears to be important. With oral or intravenous bisphosphonate therapy preceding treatment with teriparatide, there may be a delay in bone density gains, although it appears as if bone density may rise to a similar extent overall by the end of the treatment course [18]. When denosumab therapy precedes treatment with teriparatide, however, progressive or transient bone loss has been described [19].

Subcutaneous injections may not be acceptable to all patients or feasible for those with comorbidities that may affect motor function. Alternative delivery systems would be an attractive option, and there is a phase 3 trial of a transdermal abaloparatide patch (https://clinicaltrials.gov/ct2/show/NCT04064411). While it is important to consider osteoanabolic therapy for all patients at high fracture risk, antiresorptive therapy may be a better match for some patients.

Osteoanabolic therapy is well tolerated in women and men [9–12]. Hypercalcemia can occur and may prompt a reduction in calcium supplementation. In the pivotal trial of teriparatide, adverse events that were statistically greater in the teriparatide group included nausea and headache [8]. In the ACTIVE trial, hypercalcemia was less common in the abaloparatide arm compared to teriparatide; however, palpitations, nausea, and dizziness were greater in the abaloparatide compared to teriparatide and placebo arms [12]. A 15-year post-marketing surveillance study did not demonstrate an increased risk of osteosarcoma in adults treated with teriparatide [20]. While the black box warning for teriparatide to communicate serious risk was lifted by the Food and Drug Administration in January 2021, the use of teriparatide must still be avoided in patients with increased risk of osteosarcoma [4]. The black box warning for abaloparatide persists at this time.

Outcome

The patient was treated with abaloparatide 80 mcg SC daily for 18 months and recently transitioned to denosumab. Her bone density after completion of abaloparatide therapy was significant for

T-scores of −2.3 at the lumbar spine (+19.8%), −2.6 at the femoral neck, and −2.5 at the total hip (+5.3%). She has not experienced any other fractures during her treatment course. She is very satisfied with her bone density gains, and we expect further improvement with denosumab.

Clinical Pearls/Pitfalls
- Teriparatide and abaloparatide are approved osteoanabolic therapies administered as a daily subcutaneous injection.
- Osteoanabolic agents have been demonstrated to stimulate bone formation, improve bone density, and decrease vertebral and nonvertebral fracture risk.
- Osteoanabolic therapy should be considered for women and men at increased risk for fracture and for women and men with glucocorticoid-induced osteoporosis.
- Patients at high risk for fracture include those who have experienced an osteoporotic fracture, patients with very low T-scores, and patients with multiple risk factors for fracture.
- Osteoanabolic therapy must be followed by antiresorptive therapy to maintain bone density gains.
- Postmarketing surveillance has not demonstrated an increased risk of osteosarcoma in adults treated with teriparatide and the black box warning has been removed.

References

1. Silva BC, Costa AG, Cusano NE, Kousteni S, Bilezikian JP. Catabolic and anabolic actions of parathyroid hormone on the skeleton. J Endocrinol Investig. 2011;34:801–10.
2. Cusano NE, Costa AG, Silva BC, Bilezikian JP. Therapy of osteoporosis in men with teriparatide. J Osteoporos. 2011;2011:463675.
3. Tabacco G, Bilezikian JP. Osteoanabolic and dual action drugs. Br J Clin Pharmacol. 2019;85:1084–94.

4. Eli Lilly and Company. Forteo (teriparatide) [package insert]. U.S. Food and Drug Administration website. https://www.accessdata.fda.gov/drug-satfda_docs/label/2020/021318s053lbl.pdf. Accessed 15 May 2021.

5. Radius Health, Inc. Tymlos (abaloparatide) [package insert]. U.S. Food and Drug Administration website. https://www.accessdata.fda.gov/drug-satfda_docs/label/2017/208743lbl.pdf. Accessed 15 May 2021.

6. Hodsman AB, Bauer DC, Dempster DW, et al. Parathyroid hormone and teriparatide for the treatment of osteoporosis: a review of the evidence and suggested guidelines for its use. Endocr Rev. 2005;26:688–703.

7. Camacho PM, Petak SM, Binkley N, Diab DL, Eldeiry LS, et al. American Association of Clinical Endocrinologists/American College of endocrinology clinical practice guidelines for the diagnosis and treatment of postmenopausal osteoporosis-2020 update. Endocr Pract. 2020;26(Suppl 1):1–46.

8. Eastell R, Rosen CJ, Black DM, Cheung AM, Murad MH, Shoback D. Pharmacological management of osteoporosis in postmenopausal women: an Endocrine Society clinical practice guideline. J Clin Endocrinol Metab. 2019;104(5):1595–622.

9. Neer RM, Arnaud CD, Zanchetta JR, et al. Effect of parathyroid hormone (1-34) on fractures and bone mineral density in postmenopausal women with osteoporosis. N Engl J Med. 2001;344:1434–41.

10. Saag KG, Shane E, Boonen S, et al. Teriparatide or alendronate in glucocorticoid-induced osteoporosis. N Engl J Med. 2007;357:2028–39.

11. Saag KG, Zanchetta JR, Devogelaer JP, et al. Effects of teriparatide versus alendronate for treating glucocorticoid-induced osteoporosis: thirty-six-month results of a randomized, double-blind, controlled trial. Arthritis Rheum. 2009;60:3346–55.

12. Miller PD, Hattersley G, Riis BJ, et al. Effect of Abaloparatide vs Placebo on new vertebral fractures in postmenopausal women with osteoporosis: a randomized clinical trial. JAMA. 2016;316:722–33.

13. Kurland ES, Heller SL, Diamond B, et al. The importance of bisphosphonate therapy in maintaining bone mass in men after therapy with teriparatide [human parathyroid hormone(1-34)]. Osteoporos Int. 2004;15:992–7.

14. Black DM, Greenspan SL, Ensrud KE, et al. The effects of parathyroid hormone and alendronate alone or in combination in postmenopausal osteoporosis. N Engl J Med. 2003;349:1207–15.

15. Deal C, Omizo M, Schwartz EN, et al. Combination teriparatide and raloxifene therapy for postmenopausal osteoporosis: results from a 6-month double-blind placebo-controlled trial. J Bone Miner Res. 2005;20:1905–11.

16. Cosman F, Eriksen EF, Recknor C, et al. Effects of intravenous zoledronic acid plus subcutaneous teriparatide [rhPTH(1-34)] in postmenopausal osteoporosis. J Bone Miner Res. 2011;26:503–11.

17. Tsai JN, Uihlein AV, Lee H, et al. Teriparatide and denosumab, alone or combined, in women with postmenopausal osteoporosis: the DATA study randomised trial. Lancet. 2013;382:50–6.
18. Boonen S, Millisen K, Gielen E, et al. Sequential therapy in the treatment of osteoporosis. Curr Med Res Opin. 2011;27:1149–55.
19. Leder BZ, Tsai JN, Uihlein AV, et al. Denosumab and teriparatide transitions in postmenopausal osteoporosis (the DATA-Switch study): extension of a randomised controlled trial. Lancet. 2015;386:1147–55.
20. Gilsenan A, Midkiff K, Harris D, et al. Teriparatide did not increase adult osteosarcoma incidence in a 15-year US postmarketing surveillance study. J Bone Miner Res. 2021;36:244–51.

Sclerostin Inhibition

14

Cristiana Cipriani and John P. Bilezikian

Case Presentation

A 70-year-old woman had surgery for a femoral neck fracture that occurred after falling from a standing position at home. One day after admission to the orthopedic service, she underwent surgery and placement of a hip prosthesis. She recovered well without complications. A metabolic bone disease specialist was consulted for management of osteoporosis suspected to be responsible for the hip fracture.

Upon consultation, it became apparent that the patient had markedly reduced BMD when it had been measured 4 years earlier by DXA. T-scores were as follows: lumbar spine, -3.4; femoral neck, -3.6; and total hip, -3.0. She had been compliant with alendronate 70 mg weekly and vitamin D since her diagnosis. She had no history of previous clinical fragility fracture, and a recent

C. Cipriani
Department of Clinical, Internal, Anesthesiological and Cardiovascular Sciences, Sapienza University of Rome, Rome, Italy

J. P. Bilezikian (✉)
Division of Endocrinology, Vagelos College of Physicians and Surgeons, Columbia University, New York, NY, USA
e-mail: jpb2@cumc.columbia.edu

© The Author(s), under exclusive license to Springer Nature Switzerland AG 2021
N. E. Cusano (ed.), *Osteoporosis*,
https://doi.org/10.1007/978-3-030-83951-2_14

159

vertebral fracture assessment (VFA) 6 months earlier showed no evidence for vertebral fracture. The trabecular bone score (TBS) was consistent with the lowest tertile of degraded bone quality with a score of 1.13 (normal: >1.33). A systems review indicated hypothyroidism, dyslipidemia, and hypertension, for which she was on levothyroxine, a statin, and an ACE inhibitor, respectively, with good control of these comorbidities. Her maternal grandmother had sustained a hip fracture at about the same age.

A follow-up DXA exam showed the following T-score values: lumbar spine −3.2., femoral neck −3.1, and total hip −2.8, all of which showed only modest increases on alendronate therapy. The TBS was still very low and unchanged at 1.13. Laboratory evaluation excluded secondary causes of osteoporosis with all of the following tests within normal range: serum calcium, phosphorus, parathyroid hormone, 25-hydroxyvitamin D, protein electrophoresis, and celiac panel. The urinary calcium excretion was normal.

Therapy with romosozumab 210 mg monthly SC was recommended.

Assessment and Diagnosis

Osteoporosis, the most common metabolic bone disease, is characterized by reduced bone mass and microstructural deterioration, resulting in poor bone quality and reduced bone strength. These abnormalities lead to increased fracture risk. One of the underlying pathophysiologic principles that lead to osteoporosis is an imbalance between the remodeling elements of bone formation and bone resorption. This imbalance created by greater bone loss than bone gain leads, over years, to the characteristic features of reduced bone density and impaired bone quality. Advances in our understanding of basic bone biology over the past 20 years have led to new therapies for osteoporosis [1] including romosozumab, a drug that targets the Wnt signaling pathway, a major anabolic pathway for bone. Romosozumab specifically inhibits sclerostin, a molecule that helps to regulate this pathway. By inhibiting sclerostin, romosozumab enhances this osteoanabolic pathway.

The Sclerostin-Wnt Signaling Pathway

The glycoproteins that are part of the Wnt family are encoded by 19 genes in humans. They regulate growth, proliferation, survival, and function of different cells and organs [2]. Within the Wnt family, the glycoproteins that signal through β-catenin (the canonical Wnt pathway) interact with the low-density lipoprotein receptor-related protein (LRP) five or six and a seven transmembrane receptor of the Frizzled family [3]. This interaction between Wnt and these factors at the target cell facilitates the cytoplasmic phosphorylation of LRP5/6 and recruitment of axin. The complex that is eventually formed protects β-catenin from cytoplasmic phosphorylation and degradation [3]. As a result, β-catenin can gain access to the nucleus where it simulates the transcription of target genes implicated in the differentiation of mesenchymal stem cells into the osteoblastic lineage. Moreover, apoptosis of osteocytes and osteoblasts is inhibited, and osteoclastogenesis is reduced [1, 3].

Sclerostin is a glycoprotein encoded by the *SOST* gene, produced primarily by osteocytes [4]. It regulates the canonical Wnt signaling pathway by binding to the LRP5/6 complex and, thus, prevents Wnt from binding and triggering the events that result in the translocation of β-catenin into the nucleus. β-catenin is left unprotected in the cytoplasm where it undergoes phosphorylation and ultimately metabolic degradation [4]. Sclerostin, thus, acts as a brake on this pathway and helps to limit excessive bone formation. Normal skeletal homeostasis can be viewed, at least in part, as a balance between sclerostin (and other Wnt pathway inhibitors such as DKK) and Wnt.

In addition to its anti-Wnt signaling activity, sclerostin has the potential to disrupt the RANKL signaling pathway by increasing the catabolic cytokine RANKL and reducing its antagonist, osteoprotegerin, in osteoblasts. In these ways, sclerostin has the potential to both inhibit bone formation and stimulate bone resorption [5]. Sclerostin is a main regulator of bone metabolism exemplified by it anti-anabolic and pro-catabolic activities.

Sclerosteosis and Von Buchem's Disease

Clues as to how an anti-sclerostin antibody could be developed as an anabolic therapy for osteoporosis originated with the discovery of two genetic high bone mass disorders associated with loss-of-function mutations of the *SOST* gene. In the homozygous forms of sclerosteosis and Von Buchem's disease, two very rare autosomal recessive diseases, BMD is remarkably high and accrued continuously throughout life. The clinical features are hyperostosis and bone thickening that typically involve the skull, face, and jaw, with consequent prognathism, entrapment syndromes, compression of the neuronal foramina, and neurological complications [4]. Tall stature and syndactyl are also part of the phenotype [4]. In these patients, sclerostin levels are not detectable. In the heterozygous forms, in which patients have only a single mutated gene copy of the *SOST* gene, high bone mass is present without the negative clinical features of the disease. As expected, sclerostin levels in the heterozygous form of the disease are about half the level in normal individuals. In both the homozygous and heterozygous forms of these diseases, fractures do not occur [3].

With these insights, it became attractive to consider the development of an inhibiting sclerostin antibody that would facilitate the expression of the canonical Wnt signaling pathway and lead to anabolic effects on bone.

Management

Animal Models

Animal models supporting the actions of the anti-sclerostin antibody showed that this approach is associated with increased bone formation and bone mass [3].

In rat models of postmenopausal osteoporosis, treatment with an anti-sclerostin antibody resulted in a marked increase in trabecular and cortical BMD as well as improvement in bone quality as assessed by micro-computed tomography. The microstructural improvements included trabecular and cortical thickness, trabecular volume, and volumetric BMD [4, 6]. A reduction in cortical porosity was also observed [4, 6]. By histomorphometric analysis, osteoblasts are increased in number. Mineralizing surfaces are enhanced, and osteoclast surface is reduced [6]. These observations were confirmed in aged male rats and in non-human primates [3, 7–9]. Interestingly, a significant stimulation of bone formation on quiescent bone surfaces, with no increase in bone resorption markers, has been observed in male and female cynomolgus monkeys [3, 7–9]. This demonstration of enhanced bone modeling, an unusual observation in the mature human skeleton, provides another mechanism by which the anti-sclerostin antibody is anabolic. In all these studies, the inhibition of sclerostin was associated with a dose-dependent response in terms of stimulation of bone formation, increases in BMD, and improvement of bone strength and microstructure [6, 7, 10].

Animal models of bone loss from other causes, such as glucocorticoid-induced osteoporosis, immobilization, spinal cord injury, chronic inflammatory conditions, diabetes, chronic kidney disease, and multiple myeloma, were developed to investigate the effect of anti-sclerostin antibody [4, 9]. Collectively, results from preclinical studies showed that anti-sclerostin antibodies positively affect bone formation, trabecular and cortical bone mass, and strength in these conditions [4, 9].

Clinical Trials and Studies

Romosozumab is the first approved anti-sclerostin antibody for the treatment of osteoporosis. Table 14.1 shows the main characteristics of clinical trials and studies of romosozumab.

In the pivotal clinical Fracture Study in Postmenopausal Women with Osteoporosis (FRAME), an incidence of 0.5% of new vertebral fractures was observed with romosozumab vs. 1.8% in the placebo group at month 12, translating into a 73% reduction in relative risk (RR) [11]. At 12 months, BMD was 13.3% and 5.9% higher than placebo at the lumbar spine and femoral neck, respectively [11]. The design of FRAME called for a transition

Table 14.1 Characteristics of the main clinical trials and studies on romosozumab

Trial/study	Design	Primary endpoint	Inclusion criteria	Treatment arms	Number of participants
FRAME [11]	Phase 3, double-blind, placebo-controlled trial	Incidence of new vertebral fracture through 12 and 24 months	Postmenopausal women aged 55–90 Femoral neck or total hip T-score ≤ −2.5	Double-blind: monthly romosozumab 210 mg vs. placebo for 12 months Open-label: 12-month denosumab 60 mg every 6 months	Enrolled: 7180 Randomized: 3589 to romosozumab; 3591 to placebo
ARCH [12]	Phase 3, double-blind, active-comparator trial	Incidence of clinical fracture at primary analysis Incidence of new vertebral fracture through 24 months	Postmenopausal women aged 55–90 High risk for osteoporotic fracture	Double-blind: monthly romosozumab 210 mg vs. weekly alendronate 70 mg for 12 months Open-label: weekly alendronate 70 mg for 24 months	Enrolled: 4093 Randomized: 2046 to romosozumab; 2047 to alendronate
STRUCTURE [13]	Phase 3 randomized, open-label, active-comparator trial	Percentage change in total hip BMD over 12 months	Postmenopausal women aged 55–90 Oral bisphosphonate for ≥3 years (final year alendronate) Any site T-score ≤ −2.5 History of nonvertebral or vertebral fracture	Open-label: monthly romosozumab 210 mg vs. daily teriparatide 20 μg	Enrolled: 436 Randomized: 210 to romosozumab; 218 to teriparatide

Study	Design	Outcome measure	Population	Intervention	Results
McClung et al., 2018 [14]	Phase 2, placebo-controlled, parallel group study	Percentage change in BMD at months 24 and 36	Postmenopausal women aged 55–85 from previous trials; Any site T-score ≤ -2 and ≥ 3.5	Extension phase: 12-month denosumab 60 mg every 6 months vs. placebo	Enrolled: 419; 90 transitioned from romosozumab to denosumab; 90 from romosozumab to placebo
Kendler et al., 2019 [15]	Phase 2 randomized, placebo-controlled study	Percentage change in BMD at month 48	Postmenopausal women aged 55–85 from the McClung et al. study; Any site T-score ≤ -2 and ≥ 3.5	Second-course period: monthly romosozumab 210 mg	Enrolled: 167; Second course of romosozumab after placebo: 64; second course of romosozumab after denosumab: 65
BRIDGE [16]	Phase 3 randomized, placebo-controlled study	Percentage change in the lumbar spine BMD	Men aged 55–90; McClung et al. study; All site T-score at the LS, TH, or FN of ≤ -2.5 or ≤ -1.5 with a history of fragility; Nonvertebral or vertebral fracture	Double-blind: monthly romosozumab 210 mg vs. placebo for 12 months	Enrolled: 245; Randomized: 163 to romosozumab; 82 to placebo

after 12 months to alendronate in both the romosozumab and placebo arms of the trial for an additional 12 months. The group receiving romosozumab in the first year experienced a 75% reduction in RR at 24 months in comparison to the placebo group that was also transitioned to alendronate for 12 months [11].

In the second major clinical trial, the Active-Controlled Fracture Study in Postmenopausal Women with osteoporosis at high risk (ARCH), romosozumab was directly compared with alendronate for 12 months. This study did not have a placebo control group. New vertebral fractures were significantly lower with romosozumab (4%) than alendronate (6.3%) by month 12 [12]. There were also greater increases in BMD at all sites when romosozumab was compared to alendronate [12].

Like the FRAME study, the romosozumab group transitioned to alendronate after 12 months for another 12 months of therapy. The comparator alendronate group continued on alendronate for another 12 months. In the group that transitioned from romosozumab to alendronate, there were 48% and 19% RR reductions for new vertebral and nonvertebral fractures, respectively, in comparison to the alendronate-only group at 24 months [12]. The RR of hip fracture was 38% lower in the romosozumab-to-alendronate group [12]. The differences in BMD gains between the two groups were maintained for up to 36 months [12].

The third major clinical trial was an open-label, randomized, teriparatide-controlled study to evaluate the effect of treatment with romosozumab in postmenopausal women with osteoporosis previously treated with bisphosphonate therapy (STRUCTURE). In this trial, romosozumab was compared to teriparatide at 12 months. Romosozumab showed a 3.2% greater improvement in hip BMD at 12 months compared to the teriparatide group [13]. Six- and 12-month mean percentage changes in hip integral and cortical volumetric BMD, and hip strength by finite element analysis, were higher with romosozumab than teriparatide [13].

Sequential therapy with denosumab following romosozumab showed that transitioning from monthly romosozumab 210 mg for 24 months to denosumab was associated with a further increase in BMD (2.6%, 1.4%, and 1.9% at the lumbar spine, femoral neck, and total hip) compared to those who switched to placebo [14].

After 36 months, women receiving a second course of romoso-zumab, this time for only 12 months, following placebo, had 12%, 6.3%, and 6% increases at the lumbar spine, femoral neck, and total hip, respectively, from month 36 to month 48. The increase was similar to what was observed in the first 12 months of romoso-zumab [15]. In patients switching from romosozumab to placebo from month 24 to month 36, there was a reduction in BMD [15].

With much less data available in men, the placebo-controlled trial to evaluate efficacy and safety of romosozumab in men with osteoporosis (BRIDGE) trial has demonstrated that romosozumab increases lumbar spine, femoral neck, and total hip BMD [16].

Dynamics of Romosozumab on Bone Metabolism

The results from preclinical animal studies suggested early in the development of romosozumab that it was a dual action drug, with both anabolic and antiresorptive properties. Those studies showed a rapid rise in bone formation markers with return to baseline lev-els within 6 months and a rather prompt reduction in bone resorp-tion markers [1]. Since bone formation and resorption are tightly linked, an increase in bone formation would be expected to also result in an increase in bone resorption; however, with romoso-zumab, no increase in bone resorption markers is seen. This is a very different profile from teriparatide and abaloparatide in which there is a more sustained increased in bone formation markers and an eventual increase in bone resorption markers.

These observations were also appreciated with the clinical tri-als. In FRAME, serum procollagen type 1 N-terminal propeptide (P1NP) significantly increased soon after romosozumab adminis-tration, reaching a peak at 14 days; there was a simultaneous reduction in serum C-telopeptide of type 1 collagen (CTX) [11]. Similar results were observed in the ARCH trial and during a sec-ond course of romosozumab [12, 15].

As expected, in STRUCTURE, comparing romosozumab with teriparatide, serum P1NP increased in both arms, with the teripa-ratide group showing a sustained increase in comparison to the romosozumab group that showed a decline after 1 month [13]. Also in contrast were changes in the resorption marker, CTX. The teriparatide group showed the expected increase, while the romo-sozumab cohort showed a reduction in serum CTX [13].

Safety

The most discussed safety issue arising from clinical trials of romosozumab is whether there is an increase in cardiovascular events. During ARCH, serious cardiovascular events, such as cardiac ischemic and cerebrovascular events, were more frequent in the romosozumab group (2.5%) compared to the alendronate group (1.9%) [12]. In the BRIDGE trial, there was a numerical imbalance between the romosozumab (4.9%) and placebo (2.5%) groups in the rate of serious cardiovascular events [16]. Preexisting cardiovascular risk factors did not significantly influence the relative risk of such events [17]. Theoretically, this potential safety issue could be related to the expression of sclerostin in the vascular smooth muscle cells and its potential role as an inhibitor of vascular calcification [12, 17].

However, the results are controversial because ARCH did not have a placebo control. In FRAME, where there was a placebo control, no imbalance in cardiovascular events was observed. The discrepancy between these two studies has led to another hypothesis, namely, that it was not an increase in cardiovascular events in the romosozumab arm but rather a decrease in the alendronate arm. To this possibility, alendronate has appeared in some studies to have a role in protecting against cardiovascular events [18]. This possibility gains strength by noting that there were no cardiovascular events in the alendronate arm of ARCH during the first 3 months of the trial, supporting the hypothesis that alendronate may protect against cardiovascular events, at least in the short term [19]. Countering this argument are meta-analyses and other observations that alendronate was not associated with a reduction in cardiovascular events when it was administered after romosozumab [19].

Because of the uncertainty of a cardiovascular safety signal, romosozumab was approved by regulatory agencies in the USA and EU with a warning in patients suffering myocardial infarction or stroke (in the preceding year according to FDA, and at any time according to EMA).

Apart from this discussion, rates of adverse and serious adverse non-cardiovascular events were similar between treatment arms in all trials, with only mild injection-site reactions generally occurring in a higher number in the romosozumab arm [20].

Outcome

The 70-year-old woman presented in the case was referred to a specialist for further evaluation of osteoporosis, which is noteworthy because most individuals who sustain a fragility fracture of the hip are not referred for further evaluation [21]. Additionally, in this setting, such patients are at great risk for another fragility fracture. It is imperative to recognize that a fragility fracture is an event that requires urgent evaluation. Even though she had presumably been evaluated at the time alendronate was prescribed, it was appropriate to revisit the possibility of secondary causes that might have developed since.

The rationale for the specialist to recommend romosozumab is based on several compelling points. First, one could consider alendronate to have "failed" because the patient fractured and the increases in BMD were only modest. Second, romosozumab has demonstrated clear efficacy in reducing the risk of hip fracture [11, 12]. In a setting like this, moreover, one would prefer an anabolic agent that could not only improve bone density but also address the microarchitectural deterioration that she clearly demonstrated. While teriparatide is an option, romosozumab has been shown to be more effective in increasing hip BMD and several parameters of bone quality and strength [13]. Future head-to-head studies will be helpful in obtaining similar data on abaloparatide. Finally, the anabolic effect of romosozumab seems not to be blunted by previous antiresorptive therapy, as can be seen with teriparatide [13]. In women transitioning from bisphosphonate therapy, romosozumab demonstrated the same increase in BMD as patients not previously treated [13].

Clinical Pearls/Pitfalls

- Romosozumab is a recently introduced bone active agent that uniquely serves as both an anabolic and antiresorptive therapy.
- Romosozumab effectively improves bone mass and bone quality and reduces fracture risk.
- The safety profile is acceptable while controversy exists about whether there is any increase in cardiovascular risk.
- Romosozumab is an important addition to therapies in individuals with severe osteoporosis.

References

1. Bandeira L, Bilezikian JP. Novel therapies for postmenopausal osteoporosis. (1558–4410 (Electronic)).
2. Shah AD, Shoback D, Lewiecki EM. Sclerostin inhibition: a novel therapeutic approach in the treatment of osteoporosis. (1179–1411 (Print)).
3. Baron R, Kneissel M. WNT signaling in bone homeostasis and disease: from human mutations to treatments. (1546-170X (Electronic)).
4. Costa AG, Bilezikian JP. Sclerostin: therapeutic horizons based upon its actions. (1544–2241 (Electronic)).
5. Wijenayaka AR, Kogawa M, Lim HP, Bonewald LF, Findlay DM, Atkins GJ. Sclerostin stimulates osteocyte support of osteoclast activity by a RANKL-dependent pathway. (1932–6203 (Electronic)).
6. Li X, Ominsky MS, Warmington KS, Morony S, Gong J, Cao J, Gao Y, et al. Sclerostin antibody treatment increases bone formation, bone mass, and bone strength in a rat model of postmenopausal osteoporosis. (1523–4681 (Electronic)).
7. Ominsky MS, Vlasseros F, Jolette J, Smith SY, Stouch B, Doellgast G, Gong J, et al. Two doses of sclerostin antibody in cynomolgus monkeys increases bone formation, bone mineral density, and bone strength. (1523–4681 (Electronic)).
8. Ominsky MS, Niu Q-T, Li C, Li X, Ke HZ. Tissue-level mechanisms responsible for the increase in bone formation and bone volume by sclerostin antibody. (1523–4681 (Electronic)).

9. Ominsky MS, Boyce RW, Li X, Ke HZ. Effects of sclerostin antibodies in animal models of osteoporosis. (1873–2763 (Electronic)).

10. Li X, Warmington KS, Niu Q-T, Asuncion FJ, Barrero M, Grisanti M, Dwyer D, et al. Inhibition of sclerostin by monoclonal antibody increases bone formation, bone mass, and bone strength in aged male rats. (1523–4681 (Electronic)).

11. Cosman F, Crittenden DB, Adachi JD, Binkley N, Czerwinski E, Ferrari S, et al. Romosozumab treatment in postmenopausal women with osteoporosis. (1533–4406 (Electronic)).

12. Saag KG, Petersen J, Brandi ML, Karaplis AC, Lorentzon M, Thomas T, et al. Romosozumab or Alendronate for fracture prevention in women with osteoporosis. N Engl J Med. 2017;377(15):1417–27.

13. Langdahl BL, Libanati C, Crittenden DB, Bolognese MA, Brown JP, Daizadeh NS, et al. Romosozumab (sclerostin monoclonal antibody) versus teriparatide in postmenopausal women with osteoporosis transitioning from oral bisphosphonate therapy: a randomised, open-label, phase 3 trial. (1474-547X (Electronic)).

14. McClung MR, Brown JP, Diez-Perez A, Resch H, Caminis J, Meisner P, et al. Effects of 24 months of treatment with Romosozumab followed by 12 months of Denosumab or placebo in postmenopausal women with low bone mineral density: a randomized, double-blind, phase 2, parallel group study. (1523–4681 (Electronic)).

15. Kendler DA-O, Bone HG, Massari F, Gielen E, Palacios S, Maddox J, et al. Bone mineral density gains with a second 12-month course of romosozumab therapy following placebo or denosumab. (1433–2965 (Electronic)).

16. Lewiecki EM, Blicharski T, Goemaere S, Lippuner K, Meisner PD, Miller PD, et al. A phase III randomized placebo-controlled trial to evaluate efficacy and safety of Romosozumab in men with osteoporosis. (1945–7197 (Electronic)).

17. Langdahl BL, Hofbauer LC, Forfar JC. Cardiovascular safety and sclerostin inhibition - a mini-review. LID - dgab193 [pii] LID - https://doi.org/10.1210/clinem/dgab193. (1945–7197 (Electronic)).

18. Sing CW, Wong AY, Kiel DP, Cheung EY, Lam JK, Cheung TT, et al. Association of alendronate and risk of cardiovascular events in patients with hip fracture. (1523–4681 (Electronic)).

19. Cummings SR, McCulloch C. Explanations for the difference in rates of cardiovascular events in a trial of alendronate and romosozumab. (1433–2965 (Electronic)).

20. Fixen CA-O, Tunoa J. Romosozumab: a review of efficacy, safety, and cardiovascular risk. (1544–2241 (Electronic)).

21. Solomon DH, Johnston SS, Boytsov NN, McMorrow D, Lane JM, Krohn KD. Osteoporosis medication use after hip fracture in U.S. patients between 2002 and 2011. J Bone Miner Res. 2014;29:1929–37. https://doi.org/10.1002/jbmr.2202.

"Drug Holidays": When and How?

15

Priyanka Majety
and Alan Ona Malabanan

Case Presentation

A 69-year-old woman was diagnosed with osteoporosis based on BMD T-scores of −2.8 at the lumbar spine and −2.5 at the femoral neck 5 years ago and started on alendronate 70 mg weekly which she has tolerated without problem. The most recent BMD demonstrated T-scores of −1.8 at the lumbar spine and −2.0 at the femoral neck. She inquires about the possibility of discontinuing alendronate.

Assessment and Diagnosis

As of the time of this writing, there are ten FDA-approved drugs for the treatment of osteoporosis, proven to lower but not eliminate osteoporotic fracture risk. For those at highest fracture risk,

P. Majety
Division of Endocrinology, Diabetes and Metabolism, Beth Israel Deaconess Medical Center, Boston, MA, USA

A. O. Malabanan (✉)
Division of Endocrinology, Diabetes and Metabolism, Beth Israel Deaconess Medical Center, Boston, MA, USA

Harvard Medical School, Boston, MA, USA
e-mail: amalaban@bidmc.harvard.edu

© The Author(s), under exclusive license to Springer Nature Switzerland AG 2021
N. E. Cusano (ed.), *Osteoporosis*,
https://doi.org/10.1007/978-3-030-83951-2_15

one could argue for continued osteoporosis treatment paralleling the treatment of other chronic medical conditions such as hypertension, hyperlipidemia, and diabetes. However, the long persistence of bisphosphonates in bone concomitantly lowers the fracture risk and increases the risk for adverse effects, raising the possibility and need for osteoporosis drug holidays.

Bisphosphonates have a high affinity for bone hydroxyapatite and are preferentially incorporated into active bone remodeling sites. During remodeling, some bound bisphosphonate is released from bone; a portion binds again to bone and remains metabolically active. Bisphosphonates with higher affinity are more quickly rebound, increasing skeletal retention. Bisphosphonates differ in their mineral binding affinity (zoledronic acid > alendronate > ibandronate > risedronate) and their ability to inhibit farnesyl pyrophosphate synthase, which is responsible for their antiresorptive potency (zoledronic acid > risedronate > ibandronate > alendronate) [1].

Management

What Is a Drug Holiday?

The first mention of an osteoporosis drug holiday referred to bisphosphonate cessation in patients diagnosed with osteonecrosis of the jaw [2]. However, drug cessation in response to an adverse event is not truly what we consider a drug holiday now. The phrase "drug holiday," as first used by Curtis et al., means the bisphosphonate is being electively stopped temporarily, during which anti-fracture benefit might persist, while potential risks are minimized [3].

It is unusual to contemplate a drug holiday in treating chronic disease as most medications lose their effect after treatment discontinuation. But the persistence and long-term activity of bisphosphonates raise the possibility of an osteoporosis drug holiday. As detailed in Chap. 12, long-term bisphosphonate therapy is associated with adverse effects. A drug holiday allows balancing the long-term benefits with the long-term risks of bisphosphonate treatment.

Which Drugs Have Evidence for a Drug Holiday?

Drugs with Evidence Supporting a Drug Holiday: Alendronate, Zoledronic Acid, and Risedronate

In the Fracture Intervention Trial Long-term Extension Trial (FLEX), 1999 patients on 5 years of daily alendronate were randomized to alendronate (5 or 10 mg daily) or placebo for an additional 5 years. Those on 10 years of alendronate had fewer clinical vertebral fractures than those on 5 years (5.3% vs. 2.4%, respectively). Those discontinuing alendronate after 5 years had a 3.7% and 2.4% decrease in spine and hip BMD, respectively. There was no difference between the groups in morphometric vertebral or nonvertebral fractures [4]. A post hoc analysis showed that patients with T-scores of ≤ -2.5 at the femoral neck demonstrated a significant reduction in nonvertebral fractures with alendronate continuation compared with placebo (RR 0.50). No benefit was observed in patients with higher T-scores. The presence of a prevalent vertebral fracture at baseline did not interact with the demonstrated effect of femoral neck BMD on nonvertebral fracture risk [5]. A subsequent analysis noted that older age was independently associated with a greater risk of fracture (relative hazard ratio 1.54 per 5-year increase). Bone density decreases and bone turnover marker increases did not seem to predict fractures with alendronate discontinuation [6].

In an extension of the Health Outcomes and Reduced Incidence with Zoledronic Acid Once Yearly-Pivotal Fracture Trial (HORIZON-PFT), 1233 patients treated with zoledronic acid 5 mg yearly for 3 years were randomized to placebo or yearly zoledronic acid for 3 additional years. Continued treatment resulted in a 52% lower risk of morphometric vertebral fracture (fracture rates 3.0% vs. 6.2%). The risk of clinical vertebral, hip, and nonvertebral fractures did not differ between the groups [7]. A subsequent extension trial comparing those with annual zoledronic acid for 6 years with those treated annually for 9 years found minimal difference between BMD, bone turnover markers, and fracture risk, although there was a slight increase in arrhythmias in those with 9 years of treatment [8]. Recent work suggests that even infrequent dosing of zoledronic acid (5.5-year interval with zoledronic acid 5 mg) may prevent bone loss in older post-menopausal women for almost 11 years [9].

In the Vertebral Efficacy with Risedronate Therapy – North American (VERT-NA), patients treated with either daily risedronate (N = 398) or placebo (N = 361) for 3 years were followed for an additional 1 year after discontinuation. The morphometric vertebral fracture incidence remained 46% lower in the former risedronate group, as compared with the former placebo group (6.5% vs. 11.6%, respectively). However, there was no group of patients continuing on risedronate; hence, it was not possible to compare the fracture risk of discontinuing therapy with continuing therapy [10].

Drugs with Evidence Against a Drug Holiday: Calcitonin, Denosumab, Raloxifene, Estrogen, Teriparatide, Abaloparatide, and Romosozumab

Nasal calcitonin is a weak antiresorptive agent and its anti-osteoporotic effects wane quickly after discontinuing therapy. Discontinuation of calcitonin leads to increased bone turnover and bone loss [11].

Denosumab discontinuation leads to a rebound loss of antiresorptive effect and rapid BMD loss, although early studies failed to demonstrate an increase in fractures compared with placebo for up to 24 months after treatment cessation [12]. However, there have been numerous case reports of multiple spontaneous vertebral fractures occurring as soon as 7 months following denosumab cessation with one case series reporting 1 to 11 clinical vertebral fractures per patient among women treated with aromatase inhibitors for breast cancer [13]. A recent study found that denosumab discontinuers had a 3.2-fold higher overall fracture rate and a 14.6-fold higher rate of multiple vertebral fractures than those who continued denosumab [14]. A drug holiday is not recommended for denosumab. Those with prevalent vertebral fractures and longer duration of denosumab are at highest risk with discontinuation. Transition to bisphosphonate therapy is generally recommended, either with alendronate or zoledronic acid, but the optimal regimen is still a matter of ongoing research [15].

There is no residual effect for treatment with raloxifene or estrogen. With the discontinuation of raloxifene, bone turnover markers return close to baseline levels within 6 months of cessation of treatment, and all densitometric increases observed during treatment are lost within 1 year. In a study treating women with either raloxifene or conjugated equine estrogens for 5 years, discontinuation led to spine density decreases at 1 year, with inconsistent effects on hip density decrease [16]. Fracture risk changes are unclear after treatment discontinuation.

The benefits of osteoanabolic therapies are quickly lost if not followed by antiresorptive treatment. There is a rapid loss of BMD in both women and men after teriparatide cessation. Spine density declined 7.1% in women and 4.1% in men 12 months after teriparatide cessation, with total hip density declining 3.8% in women and remaining stable in men [17]. Teriparatide may now be used for more than 2 years during a patient's lifetime if there is a high fracture risk. There are no data regarding the effects on BMD or fracture risk from discontinuation of abaloparatide. Given its efficacy is dependent on PTH1 receptor binding, like teriparatide, loss of BMD is expected with abaloparatide cessation, and drug holiday is thus not recommended with abaloparatide.

Romosozumab-induced BMD gains are quickly lost with discontinuation. In a study with multiple doses of romosozumab over 24 months, discontinuation for 12 months showed a spine BMD decrease of 9.3%, although remaining above baseline, and a total hip BMD decrease by 5.4%, returning to baseline. Propeptide of type 1 collagen (P1NP) levels returned to baseline and C-telopeptide (CTX) levels rose and remained above baseline 12 months after discontinuation [18]. No fracture risk data are available for romosozumab discontinuation.

Drugs with Inconclusive/Insufficient Evidence for a Drug Holiday: Ibandronate

While ibandronate is a potent bisphosphonate, there are minimal data about the effects of ibandronate after discontinuation. However, the TRIO study extension trial suggests that spine BMD loss after 2 years of treatment and subsequently 2 years after discontinuation falls between that for alendronate and risedronate, as may be expected by its pharmacologic effects [19]. Insufficient data exist to justify a drug holiday in patients on ibandronate.

Who Is the Right Candidate for a Drug Holiday?

Patients with a low assessed fracture risk, as based on their lack of prevalent fractures, stable osteopenic BMD, non-elevated bone turnover markers, lack of increased fall risk, and lack of co-morbidities (i.e., no use of an aromatase inhibitor or glucocorticoid), following 5 years of alendronate or 3 years of zoledronic acid are ideal candidates for a drug holiday of between 3 and 5 years duration. Those who have used 3 years of risedronate may consider a shorter drug holiday of 1 year. Those initially at high risk and remaining at high risk after 5 years of alendronate or risedronate or 3 years of zoledronic acid may continue treatment for 10 years and 6 years, respectively, after which drug holiday may be reconsidered [20]. Patients with a persistently high fracture risk **_should not_** be considered for a drug holiday as the risks of interrupting therapy exceed the benefits (see Table 15.1 for details regarding risk stratification).

Lastly, ascertain the patient's reliability when considering a drug holiday. These patients need regular follow-up appointments with laboratory and BMD monitoring and adherence with adequate calcium/vitamin D intake and exercise. They will also need to communicate any significant clinical or medication changes between visits which may prompt fracture risk reassessment and reinitiation of treatment.

How Do You Monitor and Manage the Patient During a Drug Holiday? When Should the Drug Holiday End?

There are limited data guiding patient monitoring during a drug holiday or the benefits of reinitiating therapy. Discontinuation of bisphosphonate therapy leads to increases in bone turnover markers with subsequent bone loss. The FLEX and the HORIZON-PFT extension studies found no increased fracture risk related to changes in bone turnover or BMD after treatment discontinuation [6, 7]. Extension trials have suggested continued protection from

Table 15.1 Drug holiday considerations according to fracture risk

Fracture risk after treatment	Drug holiday recommendation	Example
Very high risk/prior fractures (age >70–75 years, recent fractures, frailty, glucocorticoids, T-score < −3.0, or increased fall risk, FRAX MOF > 30% or hip >4.5%)	Not recommended. Continue with total 6–10 years oral or 4–6 years IV and then reassess. Consider denosumab or anabolic therapies after treatment course if new fractures, decreasing bone density or increased fracture risk	75-year-old woman treated with alendronate for 5 years, femoral neck T-score −3.0, ongoing prednisone for rheumatoid arthritis, two prevalent vertebral fractures, last 12 months ago
High risk/prior fractures with increasing/stable BMD (femoral neck T-score > −2.5), 10-year hip fracture risk ≥3%, or risk of major osteoporotic fracture risk ≥20% and no additional fractures or risk factors	Consider drug holiday after 5 years of oral and 3 years of IV bisphosphonate therapy	70-year-old woman, menopause at age 48, lowest initial T-score −2.8, no risk factors, bisphosphonate therapy for 6 years, BMD increased over that time so lowest T-score now is −2.1
Moderate risk/no prior fractures with increasing/stable BMD (a BMD T-score at the hip and spine both above −2.5), 10-year hip fracture risk <3% or risk of major osteoporotic fractures <20% and no new fractures or risk factors	Consider drug holiday after 5 years of oral and 3 years of IV bisphosphonate therapy	68-year-old woman, menopause at age 50, initial lowest T-score −2.3, parent with a hip fracture, oral bisphosphonate treatment for 5 years, BMD stable over that time
Low risk/no prior fractures with increasing/stable BMD, a BMD T-score at the hip and spine both above −1.0, and 10-year hip fracture risk <3% and 10-year risk of major osteoporotic fractures <20%	Therapy may be discontinued and restarted when indications for treatment are met	55-year-old woman, menopause at age 52, lowest T-score −1.6, no risk factors, bisphosphonate therapy for 3 years

Table 15.2 Clinical risk factors to monitor during a drug holiday

New fracture
Smoking
Rheumatoid arthritis
Diabetes mellitus
Glucocorticoid use
Secondary causes of osteoporosis (hyperthyroidism, hyperparathyroidism, medications)
Current alcohol use (>/= 3 drinks/day)
Significant/unintentional weight loss
Initiation of new medications such as glucocorticoids, aromatase inhibitors, proton pump inhibitors, heparin, anticonvulsant therapy, SGLT2 inhibitors
Increasing fall risk

nonvertebral fractures for 1–5 years following bisphosphonate cessation [4, 7, 10].

Guidelines from the American Association of Clinical Endocrinology have recommended monitoring for fractures (clinical assessment as well as vertebral fracture assessment), clinical risk factors, BMD, and bone resorption markers [serum CTX and urine N-terminal telopeptide (NTX)] during the drug holiday. New fractures, increased fracture risk based on new clinical risk factors (i.e., aromatase inhibitors, glucocorticoids, rheumatoid arthritis, or diabetes mellitus), significant BMD decrease (i.e., greater than the least significant change for the DXA machine), or increasing CTX or NTX from baseline may prompt a discussion of ending the drug holiday and resuming treatment [21, 22]. Table 15.2 outlines the clinical risk factors to monitor during a drug holiday. Table 15.3 outlines nonpharmacologic recommendations during a drug holiday. Guidelines from the American Society for Bone and Mineral Research have suggested reassessing the drug holiday at 2–3 years for alendronate and zoledronic acid, with an earlier assessment for risedronate [20].

What Are Alternatives to a Drug Holiday?

For those who remain at high fracture risk despite therapy or who have fractures while on therapy, we cannot consider a drug holiday. Alternatives to a drug holiday include continuing osteoporosis treatment with the same medication or switching to another. The benefits and risks of continuing bisphosphonate therapy are highlighted above. Appropriate sequential medication selection requires the assessment of the patient's ongoing fracture risk, the potential for BMD increase with the alternative medication, the patient's comorbidities, and personal preferences. Readers are referred to a recent review [23]. Table 15.4 incorporates this sequential therapy data. Combination of denosumab and teriparatide may produce additional BMD gain than either denosumab or teriparatide alone over 24 months, although its effect on fracture risk reduction is not clear [24]. Combination therapy has not been approved.

Table 15.3 Recommendations during drug holiday from bisphosphonates

Maintain adequate calcium intake in diet and add supplements if needed. A total daily intake of 1200 mg/day for women age ≥50 years is recommended
Counsel patients to limit alcohol intake to no more than 2 units per day
Counsel patients to avoid or stop smoking
Counsel patients to maintain an active lifestyle, including weight-bearing, balance, and resistance exercises
Provide counseling on reducing risk of falls, particularly among the elderly. Consider referral for physical therapy, which may reduce discomfort, prevent falls, and improve quality of life

Table 15.4 Bone density effects of sequential therapies [23]

Drug		BMD effect		
Initial	Sequential	Spine	Hip	Fracture protection
Teriparatide	Raloxifene	↔	↑	?
	Alendronate	↑	↑	?
	Denosumab	↑	↑	?
Abaloparatide	Alendronate	↑	↑	↔
Romosozumab	Denosumab	↑	↑	↔
	Alendronate	↑	↑	↑
Raloxifene	Teriparatide	↑	↑	?
Alendronate	Denosumab	↑	↑	?
	Teriparatide	↑	↑	↑
	Romosozumab	↑	↑	?
Denosumab	Teriparatide	↓	↓	?

Outcome

After 5 years of alendronate, our 69-year-old female patient had an osteopenic BMD without vertebral fracture on VFA. She took adequate calcium and vitamin D and had no other risk factors for fracture. She was deemed low risk for fracture and initiated on a drug holiday. A baseline fasting, early morning CTX was ordered, with plan to repeat CTX and BMD in 1 year. She was instructed on exercise, lifestyle changes, and fall prevention. She agreed to contact us earlier if her clinical situation changed, specifically with regard to new fractures, initiation of osteotoxic medications, or the development of new health issues.

References

1. Russell RGG, Watts NB, Ebetino FH, Rogers MJ. Mechanisms of action of bisphosphonates: similarities and differences and their potential influence on clinical efficacy. Osteoporos Int J Establ Result Coop Eur Found Osteoporos Natl Osteoporos Found USA. 2008;19:733–59.
2. Marx RE, Cillo JE, Ulloa JJ. Oral bisphosphonate-induced osteonecrosis: risk factors, prediction of risk using serum CTX testing, prevention, and treatment. J Oral Maxillofac Surg. 2007;65:2397–410.
3. Curtis JR, Westfall AO, Cheng H, Delzell E, Saag KG. Risk of hip fracture after bisphosphonate discontinuation: implications for a drug holiday. Osteoporos. Int J Establ Result Coop Eur Found Osteoporos Natl Osteoporos Found. USA. 2008;19:1613–20.
4. Black DM, et al. Effects of continuing or stopping alendronate after 5 years of treatment: the Fracture Intervention Trial Long-term Extension (FLEX): a randomized trial. JAMA. 2006;296:2927.
5. Schwartz AV, et al. Efficacy of continued alendronate for fractures in women with and without prevalent vertebral fracture: the FLEX trial. J Bone Miner Res. 2010;25:976–82.
6. Bauer DC, et al. Fracture prediction after discontinuation of 4 to 5 years of Alendronate therapy: the FLEX study. JAMA Intern Med. 2014;174:1126.
7. Black DM, et al. The effect of 3 versus 6 years of Zoledronic acid treatment of osteoporosis: a randomized extension to the HORIZON-Pivotal Fracture Trial (PFT). J Bone Miner Res. 2012;27:243–54.
8. Black DM, et al. The effect of 6 versus 9 years of Zoledronic acid treatment in osteoporosis: a randomized second extension to the HORIZON-Pivotal Fracture Trial (PFT). J Bone Miner Res. 2015;30:934–44.

9. Grey A, et al. Ten years of very infrequent Zoledronate therapy in older women: an open-label extension of a randomized trial. J Clin Endocrinol Metab. 2020;105:e1641–7.

10. Watts NB, et al. Fracture risk remains reduced one year after discontinuation of risedronate. Osteoporos Int. 2008;19:365–72.

11. Overgaard K, Hansen MA, Nielsen VA, Riis BJ, Christiansen C. Discontinuous calcitonin treatment of established osteoporosis--effects of withdrawal of treatment. Am J Med. 1990;89:1–6.

12. Brown JP, et al. Discontinuation of denosumab and associated fracture incidence: analysis from the fracture reduction evaluation of Denosumab in osteoporosis every 6 months (FREEDOM) trial. J Bone Miner Res. 2013;28:746–52.

13. Gonzalez-Rodriguez E, Aubry-Rozier B, Stoll D, Zaman K, Lamy O. Sixty spontaneous vertebral fractures after denosumab discontinuation in 15 women with early-stage breast cancer under aromatase inhibitors. Breast Cancer Res Treat. 2020;179:153–9.

14. Tripto-Shkolnik L, et al. Fracture incidence after denosumab discontinuation: real-world data from a large healthcare provider. Bone. 2020;130:115150.

15. Anastasilakis AD, et al. Denosumab discontinuation and the rebound phenomenon: a narrative review. J Clin Med. 2021;10:152–79

16. Neele SJM, Evertz R, De Valk-De Roo G, Roos JC, Netelenbos JC. Effect of 1 year of discontinuation of raloxifene or estrogen therapy on bone mineral density after 5 years of treatment in healthy postmenopausal women. Bone. 2002;30:599–603.

17. Leder BZ, et al. Effects of teriparatide treatment and discontinuation in postmenopausal women and eugonadal men with osteoporosis. J Clin Endocrinol Metab. 2009;94:2915–21.

18. McClung MR, et al. Effects of 24 months of treatment with Romosozumab followed by 12 months of Denosumab or placebo in postmenopausal women with low bone mineral density: a randomized, double-blind, phase 2, parallel group study. J Bone Miner Res. 2018;33:1397–406.

19. Naylor KE, et al. Effects of discontinuing oral bisphosphonate treatments for postmenopausal osteoporosis on bone turnover markers and bone density. Osteoporos Int. 2018;29:1407–17.

20. Adler RA, et al. Managing osteoporosis in patients on long-term bisphosphonate treatment: report of a task force of the American Society for Bone and Mineral Research. J Bone Miner Res. 2016;31:16–35.

21. Camacho PM, et al. American Association of Clinical Endocrinologists and American College of endocrinology clinical practice guidelines for the diagnosis and treatment of postmenopausal osteoporosis — 2016. Endocr Pract. 2016;22:1–42.

22. Camacho PM, et al. American Association of Clinical Endocrinologists/American College of endocrinology clinical practice guidelines for the diagnosis and treatment of postmenopausal osteoporosis— 2020 update executive summary. Endocr Pract. 2020;26:564–70.

23. Langdahl B. Treatment of postmenopausal osteoporosis with bone-forming and antiresorptive treatments: combined and sequential approaches. Bone. 2020;139:115516.
24. Leder BZ, et al. Two years of Denosumab and teriparatide administration in postmenopausal women with osteoporosis (the DATA extension study): a randomized controlled trial. J Clin Endocrinol Metab. 2014;99:1694–700.

Osteoporosis Treatment Success and Failure

16

E. Michael Lewiecki

Case Presentation

A healthy and active woman who has her first measurement of BMD with DXA at age 65 years is referred for treatment. It shows T-score −3.2 at the left total hip. Vertebral fracture assessment (VFA) by DXA, performed because of historical height loss of 1.5 inches, reveals a wedge deformity at the level of T11 with 30% vertebral height loss. After being informed of the fracture, she recalls having an episode of low back pain about 1 year earlier while lifting her 2-year-old grandson. The pain resolved over several weeks without medical attention. She is started on treatment with alendronate. Two years later, a repeat DXA test shows a statistically significant BMD increase at the left total hip, with T-score improved to −2.9. Is this treatment success? She is told to continue alendronate. Three months later, she slips on spilled water on the kitchen floor, falling and fracturing her hip. Is this now treatment failure?

E. M. Lewiecki (✉)
New Mexico Clinical Research & Osteoporosis Center,
Albuquerque, NM, USA

Assessment and Diagnosis

Before starting any medication for osteoporosis, patients should be assessed for factors contributing to skeletal fragility and fracture risk. Risk factors that are correctable, such as vitamin D deficiency and poor balance, should be addressed. Patients should also be stratified by level of fracture risk considering all available clinical information, such as BMD, clinical risk factors, and/or a fracture risk algorithm (e.g., FRAX). The selection of an initial therapeutic agent can then be individualized according to the level of risk and other factors, such as patient preference, with a general theme of considering nonpharmacological therapy for those at low risk, a mild antiresorptive agent for those at moderate risk, a more potent antiresorptive agent when risk is high, and possibly an osteoanabolic agent when risk is very high. Although there is no universal consensus for defining the risk categories or the treatment options, examples (Table 16.1) are provided in recent clinical practice guidelines released by the Endocrine Society (ES) and American Association of Clinical Endocrinologists/American College of Endocrinologists (AACE/ACE) [1–3].

The patient described above has a diagnostic classification of severe osteoporosis based on an initial T-score that is −3.2 and having a vertebral fracture [4], with a risk of future fracture (27.2% 10-year probability of major osteoporotic fracture and 9.5% 10-year probability of hip fracture with FRAX) that most would consider very high [1–3]. For patients at very high risk of fracture, the ES and AACE/ACE guidelines suggest consideration of initiating treatment with an osteoanabolic agent, a bisphosphonate, or denosumab (Table 16.1).

Management

All approved treatments for osteoporosis have been shown in clinical trials to increase BMD and reduce fracture risk, but some do it better than others. As an example, denosumab increases BMD more than bisphosphonates [5–7], and some bisphosphonates may increase BMD more than other bisphosphonates [8]. Meta-regression analyses conducted by the Foundation for the National

Table 16.1 Categories of fracture risk with examples and implications for selecting initial therapy to reduce fracture risk

Level of fracture risk	Examples	Treatment considerations
Low (ES, AACE/ACE)	T-score > −1.0, and no hip or vertebral fracture, and FRAX MOF/HF < 20%/3%	Nonpharmacological
Moderate (ES)	T-score > −2.5, and no hip or vertebral fracture, and FRAX MOF/HF < 20%/3%	Nonpharmacological or bisphosphonate
High (ES, AACE/ACE)	T-score ≤ −2.5, or prior hip or vertebral fracture, or FRAX MOF/HF ≥ 20%/3%	Bisphosphonate Denosumab SERM
Very High (ES)	T-score ≤ −2.5 and fracture(s), or multiple vertebral fractures, or severe vertebral fracture (>40% vertebral height loss)	Anabolic Bisphosphonate Denosumab
Very High (AACE/ACE)	T-score < −3.0, or fracture in last 12 months, or fracture on treatment, or fracture on harmful drugs, or multiple fractures, or high fall risk, or FRAX MOF/HF > 30%/4.5%	Anabolic Bisphosphonate Denosumab

Individualizing treatment decisions according to such schemes may optimize the chances of treatment success and minimize treatment failures. Adapted from guidelines of the Endocrine Society (ES) [1, 3] and American Association of Clinical Endocrinologists/American College of Endocrinologists (AACE/ACE) [2]. *FRAX* fracture risk assessment tool, *MOF* major osteoporotic fracture, HF hip fracture, *SERM* selective estrogen receptor modulator

Institutes of Health Bone Quality Study assessed data from placebo-controlled clinical trials with many therapeutic agents. It was shown that larger BMD increases with treatment are associated with greater reductions in fracture risk [9, 10], consistent with earlier smaller studies. Osteoanabolic agents are superior to bisphosphonates in reducing fracture risk in postmenopausal women with very high baseline fracture risk [11–14]. It is now recognized that the sequence of therapy is important, with the most robust BMD response observed when treatment is started with an anabolic agent and followed with an antiresorptive medication. When anabolic therapy is given after an antiresorptive medication, there may be a delay or attenuation of the anabolic effect. Taken collectively, these data support the recommendations of the ES and AACE/ACE to use baseline fracture risk to help with the selection of the initial therapeutic agent, with osteo-anabolic therapy a consideration when fracture risk is very high.

The concept of treat-to-target (TTT) for osteoporosis [15, 16] provides some additional guidance for choosing initial therapy based on the concept that the goal of treatment is to achieve an acceptable level of fracture risk. While response to therapy is essential, it may not be sufficient in reaching an acceptable level of risk. BMD, which is a surrogate for fracture risk in untreated and treated patients, has emerged as a pragmatic treatment target with TTT for osteoporosis. For a patient who is started on treatment because of T-score $\leq$ −2.5, reaching a target BMD (e.g., T-score > −2.0) and having no recent fracture, including a morphometric vertebral fracture, can be defined as treatment success. For patients treated with denosumab, the incidence of nonvertebral fractures is lower with higher total hip T-score, with a plateau of fracture incidence with achievement of total hip T-score between −2.0 and −1.5 [17]. This suggests that aiming for T-score > −1.5, at least for denosumab, may not provide any additional anti-fracture benefit. When patients with a baseline T-score between −2.1 and −2.5 are started on treatment with denosumab, a BMD increase of at least 1.0 T-score units is associated with a decrease in fracture risk [17].

Patients treated for osteoporosis should be monitored for adherence/compliance, safety, response, and treatment success or failure. For drugs to be effective, they must be taken regularly, correctly, and for a sufficient length of time to reduce fracture risk. This is especially important for oral bisphosphonates, which have a required regimen for administration that is problematic for some patients and a poor record for compliance and persistence. Safety monitoring has many aspects, including vigilance for recognizing adverse effects of treatment (e.g., persistent thigh pain may be an early symptom of atypical femur fracture), identifying new medical conditions that could influence treatment decisions (e.g., development of chronic kidney disease may lead to discontinuation of a bisphosphonate), and listening to patients' concerns regarding fear of side effects, such as osteonecrosis of the jaw.

The outcomes of osteoporosis treatment can be categorized according to whether there is a skeletal response, treatment success, or treatment failure, with consideration of BMD, bone turnover markers, and the presence or absence of a new fracture (Table 16.2). Response to treatment is typically measured with follow-up BMD testing by DXA 1 to 2 years after starting or changing medication, and/or measurement of a bone turnover marker, such as serum C-telopeptide of type 1 collagen (CTX), a marker of bone resorption, or N-terminal propeptide type 1 procollagen (P1NP), a marker of bone formation. A significant change of a bone turnover marker may occur within several months of initiating treatment, while the time required for a significant change of BMD is much longer. Indicators of a treatment response are stabilization or a significant improvement of BMD

Table 16.2 Consequences of osteoporosis treatment

Treatment outcome	Description
Response	Stability or significant increase of BMD with appropriate change of bone turnover marker level
Success	BMD increase to T-score > −2.0 when treatment is started because of T-score ≤ −2.5, or T-score increase of at least 1.0 units when treatment is started with T-score > −2.5, and no recent fracture (e.g., within 3 years)
Failure	Two or more incident fractures; or one incident fracture with significant decrease in BMD and/or lack of appropriate change of bone turnover marker level; or significant decrease in BMD and lack of appropriate change of bone turnover marker level

Three categories of osteoporosis treatment outcomes are proposed. They are adapted from multiple published sources [9, 10, 16, 17, 19], some of which rely heavily on expert opinion, and are not necessarily mutually exclusive. In order to be a treatment success, a patient must respond to therapy; however, a patient could respond to therapy and qualify as treatment failure if there have been two or more incident fractures. Treatment success may not be achievable for some patients with medications that are currently available. Classifying patients into one or more of these somewhat arbitrary categories, when possible, may be helpful in providing a framework for consideration of further evaluation and making clinical decisions about continuing or changing therapy and a significant decrease in a bone resorption marker with antiresorptive therapy or significant increase in a bone formation marker with osteoanabolic therapy. Due to coupling of bone resorption and formation, changes in levels of markers of resorption and formation typically move in the same direction with treatment. However, romosozumab is an exception: because of its "dual effect" on bone remodeling with uncoupling of resorption and formation, bone formation markers initially increase, while resorption markers decrease. The pattern and timing of the changes in bone turnover marker levels vary with different therapeutic agents and the use of different types of bone turnover markers, with confounding of interpretation due to pre-analytical and analytical variability [18]. Therefore, the use of bone turnover markers in clinical practice may be challenging, requiring a thorough understanding of drug pharmacodynamics and familiarity with the marker that is measured. The robustness of treatment response may vary according to many factors, including patient compliance and persistence.

Assessing treatment success for an individual patient is a step beyond determining whether the patient has responded to therapy. Table 16.2 provides suggestions for identifying treatment success adapted from a report from the Working Group of the American Society for Bone and Mineral Research and the National Osteoporosis Foundation [16]; suggestions for identifying treatment failure are adapted from the Working Group of the Committee of Scientific Advisors of the International Osteoporosis Foundation [19]. Since osteoporosis is a lifelong disease and all medications lose their effectiveness when stopped (albeit with bisphosphonates losing effectiveness slower than other medications due to long skeletal retention time), treatment success should not be followed by stopping treatment; however, consideration may be given to modifying treatment when a treatment target has been reached (Table 16.3). When initial treatment has failed despite taking medication as prescribed, a thorough evaluation for contributing factors should be conducted, and a change in treatment should be considered (Table 16.3). Similarly, if monitoring shows that the patient is not on a pathway to reaching a treatment target in a reasonable period of time, consideration should be given to switching to more aggressive therapy.

Table 16.3 Responses to osteoporosis treatment success and failure

What to Do When Treatment Succeeds
If the patient has been on long-term bisphosphonate therapy (e.g., at least 5 years of an oral bisphosphonate or three annual doses of zoledronic acid), consider a bisphosphonate holiday with periodic monitoring to determine when fracture risk is once again high enough for treatment to resume. Alternatively, the bisphosphonate could be continued with a lower dose or longer dosing interval than previously.
If the patient has been on long-term denosumab (e.g., at least 5 years), consider switching to a bisphosphonate, although the ideal dose and timing for doing this is uncertain. Alternatively, continue denosumab. There are data that denosumab reduces fracture risk with a favorable safety profile for up to 10 years of continuous therapy.
If the patient is completing a course of osteoanabolic therapy, it is essential to transition to an antiresorptive medication.
If the patient is on a mild antiresorptive agent (e.g., estrogen, raloxifene), consider continuing the same medication, provided the expected benefits outweigh the possible risks.
What to Do When Treatment Fails
Replace a weaker antiresorptive agent with one that is more potent (e.g., switch from raloxifene to alendronate).
Replace an oral medication with an injectable one (e.g., switch from alendronate to zoledronic acid or denosumab).
Replace a potent antiresorptive agent with osteoanabolic therapy (e.g., switch from zoledronic acid to teriparatide, abaloparatide, or romosozumab).

These are suggestions for making treatment decisions according to the outcomes of initial treatment (i.e., whether treatment has been a success or failure)

The patient had a good response to 2 years of treatment with alendronate in terms of BMD increase (a bone turnover marker was not measured), but treatment was not fully successful because she remained at high fracture risk according to having T-score ≤ −2.5 and prior vertebral fracture [20]. It is unlikely that continuing alendronate would ever result in T-score > −2.0. In retrospect, more effective initial treatment with a greater likelihood of reaching T-score > −2.0 might have been with denosumab or an osteoanabolic agent (e.g., teriparatide, abaloparatide, romosozumab) followed by a robust antiresorptive medication.

Outcome

When the patient had a hip fracture (her second major osteoporotic fracture), it was recognized that fracture risk was even higher than previously estimated. It also raised concern about her risk of falling, triggering further assessment and interventions to optimize core strength and balance. Although the patient did not strictly meet the criteria for treatment failure presented in Table 16.2, it was recognized that fracture risk was higher than previously estimated. It was decided to switch from alendronate to an osteoanabolic agent. Although prior treatment with alendronate may delay or attenuate the bone building effects of osteoanabolic therapy, it is nevertheless likely that changing to osteoanabolic therapy will increase BMD, improve bone structure, and reduce fracture risk more than continuing alendronate. After completing a course of osteoanabolic therapy, she should be transitioned to a robust antiresorptive agent, such as denosumab, to enhance and consolidate the benefits achieved.

This patient's case reflects the complexities of managing individuals with osteoporosis and the need to consider all available clinical information when making clinical decisions. Patients do not all fit into categories described in guidelines. Treatment decisions should be individualized with consideration of the guidelines and good clinical judgment.

Clinical Pearls/Pitfalls
- Response to osteoporosis treatment is essential but not necessarily sufficient in achieving treatment success.
- Treatment success has been described as achievement of a target T-score and the absence of a recent fracture with the strategy of treat-to-target for osteoporosis.
- The occurrence of a fracture while being treated for osteoporosis is undesirable but does not necessarily represent treatment failure.

- Treatment failure has been described according to a combination of one or more fractures while on treatment, significant decrease of bone density, and lack of expected change of a bone turnover marker level.
- In the absence of consensus definitions for osteoporosis treatment success and failure, expert recommendations should be considered in the context of good clinical judgment.
- Efforts to obtain general consensus on treatment success and failure should include reaching agreement on defining acceptable levels of fracture risk and studies that evaluate changes in fracture risk associated with changing therapeutic agents.

Acknowledgments The author has received no external financial support and no assistance in the conceptualization, writing, and editing of this manuscript.

Conflict of Interest The author has received no direct income from potentially conflicting entities. His employer, New Mexico Clinical Research & Osteoporosis Center, has received research grants from Radius, Amgen, Mereo, Bindex; income for service on scientific advisory boards or consulting for Amgen, Radius; service on speakers' bureaus for Radius, Alexion; project development for University of New Mexico; and royalties from UpToDate for sections on DXA, fracture risk assessment, and prevention of osteoporosis. He is a board member of the National Osteoporosis Foundation and Osteoporosis Foundation of New Mexico. He has served on guideline committees for the International Society for Clinical Densitometry, National Osteoporosis Foundation, American Association of Clinical Endocrinologists, and North American Menopause Society.

References

1. Shoback D, Rosen CJ, Black DM, et al. Pharmacological management of osteoporosis in postmenopausal women: an Endocrine Society guideline update. J Clin Endocrinol Metab. 2020;105(3):dgaa048.
2. Camacho PM, Petak SM, Binkley N, et al. American Association of Clinical Endocrinologists/American College of Endocrinology clinical practice guidelines for the diagnosis and treatment of postmenopausal osteoporosis-2020 update. Endocr Pract. 2020;26(Suppl 1):1–46.
3. Eastell R, Rosen CJ, Black DM, et al. Pharmacological management of osteoporosis in postmenopausal women: an Endocrine Society clinical practice guideline. J Clin Endocrinol Metab. 2019;104(5):1595–622.
4. Kanis JA, on behalf of the World Health Organization Scientific Group. Assessment of osteoporosis at the primary health-care level. Technical Report.: World Health Organization Collaborating Centre for metabolic bone diseases, University of Sheffield, UK: Printed by the University of Sheffield; 2007.
5. Brown JP, Prince RL, Deal C, et al. Comparison of the effect of denosumab and alendronate on BMD and biochemical markers of bone turnover in postmenopausal women with low bone mass: a randomized, blinded, phase 3 trial. J Bone Miner Res. 2009;24(1):153–61.
6. Brown JP, Roux C, Ho PR, et al. Denosumab significantly increases bone mineral density and reduces bone turnover compared with monthly oral ibandronate and risedronate in postmenopausal women who remained at higher risk for fracture despite previous suboptimal treatment with an oral bisphosphonate. Osteoporos Int. 2014;25(7):1953–61.
7. Miller PD, Pannacciulli N, Brown JP, et al. Denosumab or Zoledronic acid in postmenopausal women with osteoporosis previously treated with oral bisphosphonates. J Clin Endocrinol Metab. 2016;101(8):3163–70.
8. Reid IR. Short-term and long-term effects of osteoporosis therapies. Nat Rev Endocrinol. 2015;11(7):418–28.
9. Bouxsein ML, Eastell R, Lui LY, et al. Change in bone density and reduction in fracture risk: a meta-regression of published trials. J Bone Miner Res. 2019;34(4):632–42.
10. Black DM, Bauer DC, Vittinghoff E, et al. Treatment-related changes in bone mineral density as a surrogate biomarker for fracture risk reduction: meta-regression analyses of individual patient data from multiple randomised controlled trials. Lancet Diabetes Endocrinol. 2020;8(8): 672–82.
11. Saag KG, Petersen J, Brandi ML, et al. Romosozumab or Alendronate for fracture prevention in women with osteoporosis. N Engl J Med. 2017;377(15):1417–27.

12. Saag KG, Shane E, Boonen S, et al. Teriparatide or alendronate in glucocorticoid-induced osteoporosis. N Engl J Med. 2007;357(20): 2028–39.
13. Hadji P, Zanchetta JR, Russo L, et al. The effect of teriparatide compared with risedronate on reduction of back pain in postmenopausal women with osteoporotic vertebral fractures. Osteoporos Int. 2012;23(8): 2141–50.
14. Kendler DL, Marin F, Zerbini CAF, et al. Effects of teriparatide and risedronate on new fractures in post-menopausal women with severe osteoporosis (VERO): a multicentre, double-blind, double-dummy, randomised controlled trial. Lancet. 2018;391(10117):230–40.
15. Lewiecki EM, Kendler DL, Davison KS, et al. Western osteoporosis alliance clinical practice series: treat-to-target for osteoporosis. Am J Med. 2019;132(11):e771–e7.
16. Cummings SR, Cosman F, Lewiecki EM, et al. Goal-directed treatment for osteoporosis: a progress report from the ASBMR-NOF Working Group on goal-directed treatment for osteoporosis. J Bone Miner Res. 2017;32(1):3–10.
17. Ferrari S, Libanati C, Lin CJF, et al. Relationship between bone mineral density T-score and nonvertebral fracture risk over 10 years of Denosumab treatment. J Bone Miner Res. 2019;34(6):1033–40.
18. Naylor K, Eastell R. Bone turnover markers: use in osteoporosis. Nat Rev Rheumatol. 2012;8(7):379–89.
19. Diez-Perez A, Adachi JD, Agnusdei D, et al. Treatment failure in osteoporosis. Osteoporos Int. 2012;23:2769–74.
20. Adler RA, El-Hajj Fuleihan G, Bauer DC, et al. Managing osteoporosis in patients on long-term bisphosphonate treatment: report of a Task Force of the American Society for Bone and Mineral Research. J Bone Miner Res. 2016;31(1):16–35.

Index

© The Editor(s) (if applicable) and The Author(s), under exclusive   197
license to Springer Nature Switzerland AG 2021
N. E. Cusano (ed.), *Osteoporosis*,
https://doi.org/10.1007/978-3-030-83951-2